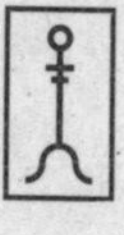

D1024122

Elliot J. Krane, M.D.

Director, Pain Therapeutics
Lucile Packard Children's Hospital
Stanford University Medical Center

with Deborah Mitchell

A Fireside Book
Published by Simon & Schuster
New York London Toronto Sydney

Relieve Your Child's Chronic Pain

A Doctor's Program for Easing Headaches, Abdominal Pain, Fibromyalgia, Juvenile Rheumatoid Arthritis, and More

A LYNN SONBERG BOOK

DISCLAIMER

This publication contains the opinions and ideas of its author. It is intended to provide helpful and informative material on the subjects addressed in the publication. It is sold with the understanding that the author and publisher are not engaged in rendering medical, health, or any other kind of personal professional services in the book. The reader should consult with his or her medical, health or other competent professional before adopting any of the suggestions in this book or drawing inferences from it.

The author, publisher, and proprietor specifically disclaim all responsibility for any liability, loss or risk, personal or otherwise, which is incurred as a consequence, directly or indirectly, of the use and application of any of the contents of this book.

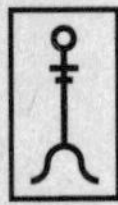

FIRESIDE
Rockefeller Center
1230 Avenue of the Americas
New York, NY 10020

For information regarding special discounts for bulk purchases,
please contact Simon & Schuster Special Sales at 1-800-456-6798
or business@simonandschuster.com

Designed by William Ruoto

Manufactured in the United States of America

10 9 8 7 6 5 4 3 2 1

Library of Congress Cataloging-in-Publication
Data Control Number: 2004058955

ISBN 0-7432-6203-4

Contents

Introduction

One night when my son Zach was four, I came home from a late night meeting at the hospital, and my wife told me Zach had hurt his elbow in the playground that day. I went to his bedroom to see him and give my sleeping son a kiss before I went to bed, and in a glance I could see his elbow was broken. My heart sank. My perfect little boy was now broken, and I could imagine the pain he experienced and would experience for several more days.

In Zach's case, as upset as I was by his injury and suffering, I knew that in a few days it would be over and his bones would heal strongly and painlessly. But the overwhelming feelings that I felt, and that any parent would experience in a similar circumstance, pale in comparison to the unending feelings of grief, loss, frustration, depression, and hopelessness that parents feel when the most precious thing in their lives, their children, suffer from pain that is chronic, pain that is unrelenting, or pain that keeps coming back over and over again, and doctors do not know what to do.

Unfortunately, we cannot always be successful in eliminating chronic pain, but we can be and are always successful in minimizing the pain, in teaching children and parents how to live and function with some pain, and most importantly of all, in eliminating suffering, for it is the suffering that makes pain unbearable, not the pain itself.

How many children experience chronic pain? Most people are astounded when they hear that up to 14 million people younger than eighteen in this country live with such pain, according to the American Pain Society. Unfortunately, these figures are not news to me. As director of an interdisciplinary pain management clinic at the Lucile Packard Children's Hospital at Stanford University in Palo Alto, California, and professor of pediatrics and professor of anesthesia at Stanford University School of Medicine, I see the reality of childhood chronic pain firsthand. And, if you are reading this book, you do, too, and you want to know what you can do to help ease the suffering. This book can help you.

How to Use This Book

This book is divided into three parts: the second part builds on the first, and the third brings together thoughts and concepts from the first two. Understanding chronic pain in children is baffling for many parents, so in Part I, I help you understand its unique features; how it differs from adult pain; and how we recognize, measure, and evaluate it. In this section I also explain the most common types of chronic pain and share some patients' stories. Along the way, there are cross-references to subsequent chapters for detailed information on treatment options for the various chronic pain conditions.

Part II, "A Program to Treat Your Child's Chronic Pain," is the nuts and bolts of the book. Here, in six chapters, you will learn about the many options for alleviating your child's pain, beginning with guidelines on how to find the most competent pain professionals, treatment facilities, and support. This is followed by several chapters on effective therapies, including mind-body techniques and physically based therapies, which include guidelines you can adapt at home; and the use of medications and other medical modalities that have proved effective. Because the success of any program to treat childhood chronic pain partly depends on ensuring your child has a healthy family, social, and educational environment, in Part II you will also learn about the impact of stress on the hurting child and family members and how to cope with it and the emotions it stirs up. Finally in this section you will also learn how to help your child thrive outside the home and interact with schoolmates, teachers, friends, and others in his or her environment.

In Part III, I have brought together some of the questions parents ask about their child's pain, plus several stories of how young people have triumphed over their pain challenges. I've called this section "Bringing Back the Laughter" because there's nothing as beautiful as the music of a child's laughter. And at my clinic, our goal is to bring that laughter back.

I hope this book will be a first step toward that laughter for you, the many mothers and fathers whose children are afflicted by chronic pain, by helping you to understand why pain occurs, how it can be treated, by whom it can be treated, and how suffering can be alleviated.

Finally, this book is dedicated to my great teachers in this field, the late Dr. John Bonica, upon whose thinking and skills the entire field of pain management was founded, and his able and insightful successor at the University of Washington, Dr. John Loeser. But as great as these professional mentors and professors were, my greatest teachers have been children themselves, who as my patients have taught me to differentiate what is important from what is not.

Part I

Children and Pain

Chapter 1

UNDERSTANDING YOUR CHILD'S PAIN

As a parent or grandparent, it is unimaginably difficult to watch a child suffer, to want to relieve the pain but not know where to turn or what approach to use. Your frustration and anger, anxiety and fear are understandable. Yet these very human emotions, which are displays of your love and concern, can get in the way of the very goal you wish to achieve: to relieve your child's pain and suffering. While health-care practitioners are usually successful at relieving acute pain—a burst appendix, a broken arm, an abscessed tooth—the same can't be said about chronic pain. If your child experiences chronic pain, you're probably feeling all the emotions we just mentioned.

The good news is, you can channel those emotions into positive, effective actions that can help you help your child. That's what this book is about: showing you how you can encourage your child to live his or her life to the fullest, with as little pain and discomfort as possible.

My decades of experience in working with children who live with chronic pain have shown me that even with the worst cases of childhood pain, we can still make a positive difference in the lives of these children and help make their childhood experience a more positive one. To make that difference, there are three main things you, as parents, need to do:

- understand the unique nature of childhood pain
- know where and how to get competent help for your child's pain
- have a comprehensive understanding of all the treatment options available to you

I firmly believe that in order for people to overcome an obstacle or beat an opponent, it's necessary to understand what they are up against. Childhood pain can be a formidable opponent, but armed with the proper tools, you can learn how to combat it and teach your child to have some control over it. In this chapter and the next, we explore the features of childhood pain so you will have a clear understanding of how pain works in young people. Be prepared to put aside some or all of your preconceived notions about childhood pain, and enter the world of childhood once again.

HOW COMMON IS CHILDHOOD PAIN?

It's a fact of life: children get hurt, and they experience pain. They run through the house, jump off the furniture, tumble down stairs, fall off their bikes, and generally barrel through life. Along the way, they get cuts and bruises, sprains and strains, and sometimes a broken bone or worse. They also tend to experience bouts of minor medical problems, such as colds, flu, and earaches. In fact, during a one-month period, a normal, healthy child experiences about four acute painful events. *Acute* means the pain is short-lived and usually can be identified and described easily.

Thus, if your ten-year-old daughter has a tooth pulled, she can expect to feel throbbing pain after the Novocain wears off and will likely need to take ibuprofen for a day or two until the pain subsides. If your three-year-old son has his tonsils removed, he will experience postoperative pain for several days, which will be treated with painkillers and plenty of ice cream. And when your eight-year-old takes a bad fall from his skateboard and breaks his arm, the arm will likely heal nicely once it's set in a cast, and your child will quickly go about his usual activities, with some limitations for a while, but also proudly displaying his "badge of honor."

Children can also experience a more persistent or long-term type of pain. In fact, for an estimated 10 million children, pain is *chronic* or *recurrent,* which means it lasts for extended periods of time or recurs at regular or irregular intervals. (For the sake of simplicity, we will use the term "chronic pain" to describe both chronic and recurrent pain unless "recurrent" is specifically meant.) In otherwise healthy children, and in girls more often than in boys, recurring headache or migraine, abdominal pain, or limb pain can occur several times a week. The pain usually is not associated with a disease or other medical condition, but it is very real and can be debilitating. Other types of chronic pain in children can include facial pain, back pain, cancer pain, fibromyalgia, and others, which we discuss in depth in Chapter 2. (See "Pain in a Nutshell.")

Regardless of the source of or reason for chronic pain, it usually has a dramatic impact on children's lives and can cause them to miss school, sports events, family activities, and play time with friends. It has negative effects on their relationship with their parents, siblings, and friends, and can cause them to become depressed, withdrawn, fearful, and anxious.

PAIN IN A NUTSHELL

PAIN occurs when special nerve endings, called nociceptors, are activated by injury, trauma, or illness, such as an acute or chronic disease, excessive cold or heat, or chemical changes in the body's tissues. When they are activated, they transmit pain messages to the brain.

SOMATIC PAIN is pain that is the result of normal processing of stimuli that can or does damage normal tissues. Examples include cuts, punctures, sprains, abrasions, inflammation (from infection or an arthritis-type condition), bone fractures, burns, and obstructions (e.g., an obstructed bowel). Somatic pain typically lasts for a limited amount of time: once the damaged tissue heals, the pain goes away. Arthritis pain is an exception. Somatic pain also usually responds well to opiods.*

NEUROPATHIC PAIN is pain that results from a malfunction or injury in the nervous system. Although the pain is usually triggered by an injury, the injury may or may not involved damage to the nervous system. The pain persists for months or years because the pain signals continue to be sent to the brain, long after any damaged tissue has healed. Neuropathic pain is stubborn; it doesn't respond as well to standard pain killers as does somatic pain, although it often responds to antidepressants and anticonvulsant medications. Examples of neuropathic pain include complex regional pain syndrome and some components of cancer pain.

COMBINED PAIN occurs in some conditions that have characteristics of both types of pain. One example that is relevant to childhood pain is migraine.

In short, chronic pain can rob a child of her childhood and have a permanent effect on how she deals with pain as an adult. It can change a child's life if the pain and the child's relationship with it are not handled effectively. The good news for you as a parent is that you and your child can learn how to manage and treat pain in ways that will result in a more fulfilling and comfortable life.

WHAT'S UNIQUE ABOUT CHILDHOOD PAIN

Humans are complex beings, and the experience of pain is not the same for people of all ages. Researchers now accept that young people—from the fetal stage through adolescence—experience pain differently than do adults. There are several reasons why a child's pain is different from and in some ways unique when compared with adult pain. Understanding these differences and special features can help you better understand your child's pain and thus make you better able to manage it and help your child. Let's look at those differences.

---

* The word "opiate" refers to a drug (such as morphine) that is derived from opium from the poppy plant, while the word "opioid" is such a drug or is one that is chemically similar to drugs derived from opium. I prefer the word "opioid" to the word "narcotic" to describe these powerful painkillers, a group that includes codeine, hydrocodone, oxycodone, morphine, hydromorphone, and fentanyl. This is because "narcotic" carries a very negative and legal connotation in our society, and because the word itself is a misnomer. "Narcotic" is derived from the Greek word *narcos,* meaning "sleep." The purpose of prescribing opioid painkillers is not to produce sleep but to produce pain relief.

Your son or daughter may be the spitting image of you, yet it's important to remember that children are not little adults and they are not you in a pint-sized version. That means their experiences with pain aren't miniature either, but they *are* different. To help you understand why your young children react to painful experiences the way they do, let's look at what's unique about childhood pain and some of the factors that contribute to how they experience and respond to pain.

Kids Experience and Express Pain Differently Than Adults

As adults, we are at an advantage when it comes to our relationship with pain. For one thing, we have a working definition—"unpleasant sensory and emotional experience associated with actual or potential tissue damage or described in terms of such damage," according to the International Association for the Study of Pain—which gives us an intellectual understanding of pain. Such a definition means nothing to young children, although older teens may appreciate its meaning.

As adults, we have past experiences with pain that we can use as points of reference; for example, we know that a paper cut is just a minor irritation, while slicing a finger down to the bone is much more serious, and we know how to react appropriately in each case. Yet young children may cry equally loudly if these situations were to happen to them.

As adults we also know that pain can usually be treated successfully with drugs or an alternative approach. That is, because we have a vast store of reference, we know there is an end in sight. Young children, however, only know the moment, and imagine the pain will go on forever. The younger the child, the smaller his or her frame of reference, and so the fear of endless pain is more real.

So if a three-year-old cuts her finger and she is hurting, she doesn't have the capacity to understand that the pain is temporary, that the pain from the cut will fade quickly, and that in ten minutes she will likely be back playing again. She only knows that it hurts NOW, and her blood-curdling screams are not indicative of the seriousness of the injury, just how serious it is to her. Perhaps you can remember a painful injury or incident you had as a child and how you felt. If you can't, be assured that your perspective of pain was different then than it is now.

The bottom line is, children experience and express pain differently than adults because they have an entirely different frame of reference. One of the most obvious—and most significant—factors in that frame of reference is age.

Age: Preschool. Children's attitudes toward, perceptions of, and responses to pain change as they get older. Each and every time children experience discomfort or pain, they add the memory of the event to their databank of information. This doesn't mean they always understand the information they are gathering, but it is still added to the mix. These memories are important because they have a great impact on how children cope with pain for the rest of their lives.

Beginning around two years of age, children can verbalize their experiences with pain, often using words like "boo-boo" or "ouchie." (Before age two, parents and doctors must rely solely on how children look, sound, and react to get an idea of how serious pain is. We talk about how we measure pain in Chapter 2 under "How Childhood Pain Is Rated.")

At this age and up to about age six, children are learning about pain and what it means. Generally they are fascinated with any visible evidence of pain, such as scars, black and blue marks, scabs, and stitches. All wounds, big and small, are significant to them, yet it is the accumulated knowledge they gather from these types of events that will help them describe and quantify pain as they grow older. You'll see why this is important when, later in this chapter, we talk about how we measure pain in children.

Preschoolers are also learning about cause and effect. When a three-year-old child rides his tricycle over a bump, falls off the bike, and hits his head (while wearing a helmet, of course!), he will likely associate the pain with hitting his head and not the fact that he hit an obstacle that caused the fall. However, he is beginning to find reasons for his pain. While children can grasp the cause and effect associated with acute pain (if you play with matches, you can get burned; if you run too fast you can fall and get hurt; if you fall out of a tree you can break your leg), it can be a very difficult concept when it comes to chronic pain. We talk about how to talk to your child about chronic pain in Chapter 8.

Preschoolers also think that their parents, grandparents, and other authority figures know exactly what hurts and how much, and that they can automatically fix it. This may be true for a bruise, a smashed finger, or a cut on the knee. These acute, painful experiences are easy to see and the pain they cause usually fades quickly on its own. However, the pain may disappear even faster when mommy says "Let mommy kiss it and make it better" and offers a cookie or the promise of a video.

But once again, when the pain is chronic, and especially invisible (e.g., a migraine, abdominal pain, chronic ear pain), preschool children cannot understand what's happening. They want to know: "Why can't mommy make it go away with kisses and cookies?" "Why can't I see my boo-boo?" (See Chapter 8, in the section "Why Do I Hurt? Talking to Your Child about Pain," for help with your child's questions about pain.)

Age: Elementary School. Beginning around age seven, children are better able to both verbalize their feelings of pain and understand why pain happens. They may also realize that chronic pain may be associated with something serious, and this may frighten them, cause undue stress, and thus ultimately make their pain worse. (We talk about pain, stress, and how parents can help their child deal with these issues in Chapter 7.)

Elementary school–age children are also capable of assigning emotions and feelings to their pain. Take nine-year-old Christopher, for example. His mother brought him into the clinic because he had been experiencing recurring headaches. When asked if he could tell me where his head hurt, he pointed to the right side of his head with a circular motion. "It's like somebody is inside my head with a boom box," he said. When asked how getting these headaches affected his life, he said, "I get real mad because I can't play basketball with my friends. It hurts too bad. And sometimes I throw up. I wish they'd stop." But when I addressed these same questions to four-year-old Paulina, she hid her face in her mother's shirt and wouldn't look at me.

Age: Teen Years. Children twelve years and older have had more opportunities to experience different types and levels of pain, so they typically can better explain how they feel. They also usually have very emotional responses to pain. One reason for this emotional response is that adolescence is inherently a highly charged time of life. Chronic pain is an intrusion into their lives: their quest for independence and a break from parental control, and their desire to belong to a group and to be accepted. Teenagers who experience chronic pain feel they have no control during a time when control is so vitally important to them.

These issues can be extremely stressful for teenagers. Stress can not only compound their pain but also contribute to depression, which is a common occurrence among adolescents. Stress and depression are addressed in more depth in Chapter 7.

How Parents and Other Adults Respond. Parents play a critical and unique role in the relief, or continuance, of their child's pain. For one thing, children turn to their parents for guidance on how to react to a painful experience. Parents who dismiss painful events by saying things like "It's nothing to worry about," or "Don't be such a baby," or "Nothing's wrong with you" may be sending the message that the pain isn't real or important or that the parent doesn't believe the child.

When children have acute pain, it's common for parents to nurture them until the hurt heals. When nine-year-old Stephen had the flu, his mother let him lie on the couch and watch videos while she brought him juice and soup. When eleven-year-old Charisa broke her leg, she got the "royal treatment" from her parents and sisters for about a week until she was able to master her walking cast and crutches. The entire time eight-year-old Joel had strep throat, he didn't have to do his chores, and his mother bought him all his favorite desserts. You can probably add some spoiling routines to this list. Face it, we like to pamper our kids when they don't feel well. This is a very appropriate response to an acute, short-lived injury or illness, but it is often counterproductive and maladaptive when chronic pain is involved.

If you spoil your child who has chronic pain, you may be sentencing him or her to a life on the couch or on the sidelines. Instead of the message being "I care about you so I'm going to do everything for you," the message is "You're sick and you can't do anything for yourself," or "You're not okay," or "Give up."

Children who live with chronic pain need caring and supportive role models, and most often they turn to their parents. In this book we are going to show you how to acquire and provide that support.

Gender. For a variety of possible reasons, boys and girls may differ in how they perceive pain, express it, and cope with it. Overall, girls tend to rate more procedures (e.g., having a tooth pulled, setting a fractured bone) as painful than do boys. Girls also tend to be more anxious, nervous, or fearful about pain, while boys are usually angry. At least one reason for these differences is cultural. Generally, when girls experience pain they are encouraged to take medication, to lie down, or to relax. Boys, however, are usually expected to "tough it out," to "take it like a man," even though the level of pain a girl and a boy may be experiencing is the same. Thus the messages girls and boys get from authority figures—parents, grandparents, teachers, coaches—regarding pain as they grow up impacts how they perceive, express, and manage pain.

Attitude. Children are attuned to how their parents and other authority figures feel about their health conditions. If you've been taking your child to different doctors or you've been trying different medications and the results haven't been satisfactory, it's important that you don't reflect a defeated or negative attitude. If you, the child's authority figure, feel helpless and hopeless, how else can you expect your child to feel? One thing that can help your attitude is to understand as much as you can about your child's pain and any of the ways it can be treated. That's what this book is here to do.

Sense of Control. When you feel out of control or you feel as though the outcome of a situation is out of your hands, it's natural to feel stressed, anxious, afraid, and helpless. If you feel this way, can you imagine how children feel under similar circumstances? But there are things we can do to reduce the levels of these feelings and, in some cases, also reduce the amount of pain children experience. It all boils down to giving children some control over or some say in the painful situation.

Naturally, the amount of control any child can have over a painful event depends on several factors, including age, the seriousness of the condition or event, and what the treatment or procedure is. Yet even the simplest activity may prove helpful. When thirteen-year-old Bryan began to experience frequent headaches and nausea, he was very frustrated about missing soccer games after school and often not being able to listen to music with his friends. His sense of helplessness and frustration was only making his head pain worse. He told his father that "I feel like the headaches control me."

Bryan had medication he could take when the headaches were bad, but he needed something that gave him more hands-on control. To help reduce his feeling of helplessness, Bryan was shown some simple techniques he could use whenever he felt stressed or when a headache was coming on. Bryan found that knowing which pressure points to massage and how to do deep breathing exercises and progressive relaxation helped him feel more in control of his head pain. (More about these and other techniques in Chapters 4 and 5.)

Kids Experience a Greater Diversity of Chronic Pain Than Adults

Generally, chronic pain in adults most commonly falls into one of several categories: back pain (the number one complaint by far in any pain clinic), migraine, myofascial pain (for example, fibromyalgia), and joint pain (most frequently osteoarthritis). Chronic pain in children, however, tends to fall into different classes. On the one hand are those chronic pain syndromes that are functional, meaning they are not associated with any tissue or organic injury. These include headache, migraine, recurrent abdominal pain (which typically includes cyclic vomiting and irritable bowel syndrome), limb pain (which includes complex regional pain syndrome type 1), and fibromyalgia.

On the other hand are chronic and recurrent pain syndromes associated with many diseases, such as juvenile rheumatoid arthritis and other collagen vascular diseases (which are more common in children than they are in adults), sickle cell anemia, human immunodeficiency virus/acquired immunodeficiency syndrome (HIV/AIDS), and cystic fibrosis. We discuss all of these chronic pain conditions in Chapter 2.

Kids Respond Differently to Mind/Body Therapy and Drugs

One hundred percent of the children who are treated at our pain clinic get one or more forms of complementary treatment at least once, and most of them continue with these therapies. Why? There are several reasons, but primarily because they are very effective in children. As you'll read about later in the chapters on "Using the Power of the Mind" and "Tapping into the Body's Healing Powers," children are often more accepting of alternative or complementary therapies than adults, as they have few if any preconceived ideas about these practices. They also typically have active imaginations, which makes working with methods such as visualization/guided imagery, self-hypnosis, and play therapy not only beneficial but fun as well.

When it comes to medications, children respond differently to drugs than older individuals. We discuss this issue in more depth in Chapter 6, "When Medications are Needed," but for now let's remember that children are not miniature adults: you can't just give them a lesser dose of a drug and expect it to work the same way it does in an adult. Children may have a different response not only in terms of how much relief they get from the drug, but also in the type and severity of side effects from the medications.

TREATING CHILDHOOD PAIN: WHAT'S THE GOAL?

When it comes to treating pain in children, the approach and goals differ depending on whether we are treating acute or chronic pain. In acute pain, the goal is to eliminate or significantly reduce the pain, which we do more often with drugs. Because the pain associated with an acute condition is only temporary, the use of drugs is typically not something about which parents should worry. In the majority of cases, children need to take a few doses, or perhaps even a week or two of medication, after which the pain will be gone and the treatment will be finished. This is how we usually treat, for example, an earache, sore throat, headache, and muscle pain from the flu.

When you're treating chronic pain, treatment is typically administered over months, and for some children, years or a lifetime. Whenever possible, I keep use of medication to a minimum to help avoid side effects and drug tolerance. Fortunately, children generally respond very well to mind-body techniques, which means in many cases minimal or no drugs are needed for pain management.

In children who have chronic pain, we want to eliminate or minimize the pain, yet this is not always easy and it isn't always the goal. In children who can expect to experience a lifetime of pain, the implication is that they will need to take medications for the rest of their lives. Physiologically and financially, this may not be the best approach to take. Drug tolerance (reaching a point where higher and higher doses are needed to achieve the same results) and side effects can both be significant problems when treating chronic pain.

That's why when I evaluate a child for treatment, I am mindful of the goals of the management of chronic pain, which are to restore or maximize the child's level of functioning and to reintegrate the child into his or her normal life as much as possible. And while I don't necessarily shy away from the use of pharmaceuticals to manage chronic pain, it is not the first tool I pull out of my treatment box. Often the use of medications impairs children's functioning by making them sleepy, unable to concentrate, or sluggish. That's why I am thankful there are many other pain management approaches we can use to achieve our goals, and that children typically respond to them very well. We talk about those approaches in Chapters 4–7 in Part 2.

WHY IT'S IMPORTANT TO TREAT CHILDHOOD PAIN

The obvious response to this statement is, "Of course, so my child won't suffer; so he or she can be as happy as possible and live as painless a life as possible," and that is certainly the most important reason. Yet there is another reason as well, one about which researchers are learning more and more. That is, that chronic pain experienced during childhood may predispose individuals to more debilitating pain later in life; in other words, pain begets pain. This is because chronic pain changes the way the central nervous system processes and transmits pain nerve signals, making it more sensitive to stimulation over time. If we can identify and successfully treat childhood pain, then we will be able to reduce or even eliminate problems later in childhood and adulthood.

In fact, researchers suspect that when premature infants experience recurring, painful procedures, as are sometimes necessary to ensure the survival of such infants, the procedures may damage their nerve cells. Thus hyperstimulation of the nerves may result in long-term consequences to the nervous system. We are not yet certain how significant those consequences may be. This question is a subject of a Food and Drug Administration and National Institutes of Health task force that is looking at pain control in newborns.

BOTTOM LINE

While adults have a more pragmatic approach to pain, a child's pain is layered: there's the biological/physical layer, and there's the very influential layer composed of emotions, thoughts, physical skills, behaviors, and cognitive processing abilities. The composition of this other layer has a significant impact on how a child experiences and expresses pain. Parents need to view their child's pain with different eyes—with the eyes of the child they once were—and so hopefully will better understand and be better able to help their child meet the challenge.

In the next chapter I will take you on a more intimate trip into the world of childhood chronic pain. As a parent you are already somewhat familiar with the road you've been traveling, but it's my hope to make the journey a little easier by sharing what health-care practitioners, parents, and children with chronic pain know about the challenges.

Chapter 2

WHAT HURTS: CHRONIC PAIN SYNDROMES OF CHILDHOOD

At any given moment, approximately 10 million children in the United States are living with chronic pain. This number is hard for many people to fathom or even believe. What conditions are so many children suffering from? And, most important, what can be done to alleviate or eliminate their suffering? These are the questions we address in this chapter.

If you are the parent of a child who experiences chronic pain, this chapter can help you better understand the medical condition or disease that is at the root of that pain. I believe it is important for parents to understand the factors that are responsible for their child's suffering, because then they are often better able to cope with the situation (living with a child who has chronic pain is typically very stressful for all family members—the hurting child, the parents, and any siblings) and explain the pain to the child and any brothers and sisters. Most important, they are better equipped to help the child manage the pain and live as full and childlike a life as possible.

I'll first briefly describe how we rate childhood pain, and then discuss in depth the most common causes of pain in children. As each of the more common causes of chronic pain in children in this chapter is described, I'll also offer management and treatment options and refer you to the appropriate chapters in Part 2 of this book to learn more about them and how you can incorporate them into your child's life where relevant. It is my hope that a more thorough understanding of the condition that affects your child can do much to ease both physical and emotional pain, as well as your anxiety and concerns.

HOW CHILDHOOD PAIN IS RATED

If you go to your doctor complaining of muscle pain or headache, you can rate the pain using words such as piercing, throbbing, or sharp; or you can rate it from 0 to 10, with 0 being no pain and 10 being the worst pain you have ever felt. You can make these ratings because you have life experience, points of reference, and a vocabulary that allow you to do so. A young child cannot communicate his or her pain to you in words or numbers. Older children can count but often will not have the points of reference or experience to communicate the severity of pain.

When you take your hurting child to a health-care practitioner, you can expect him or her to somehow identify the severity of your child's pain. Rating a child's pain is a step other physicians and I use when we evaluate a child's level of pain, but I don't think the scales we use are very useful for parents because the observations we make are open to interpretation. However, I want to briefly explain the methods we use so you will understand how and when they are helpful and why they are sometimes not.

Infants to Three Years

For children who are younger than thirty-six months, as well as those older children who are nonverbal, for example who have cerebral palsy, there are several scales that allow doctors to rate the severity of pain. With the FLACC scale (Face, Legs, Activity, Cry, Consolability), for example, we look at the child and rate his or her appearance or response from 0 to 2 on each of five factors, with 0 indicating a normal appearance or response and 2 abnormal. For example:

	0	1	2
Face	No expression	Occasional frown or grimace	Frequent to constant frown
Legs	Relaxed	Uneasy/restless	Kicking or legs drawn up
Activity	Lying quietly, moves easily	Squirming, tense	Arched, rigid or jerky
Cry	No crying	Whimpers or moans	Screams, sobs, or cries steadily
Consolability	Content, relaxes	Reassured by talking, hugging	Difficult to comfort

The Riley Infant Pain Scale approaches pain in a similar way, rating six factors ranging from optimal (second column) to worst (last column):

	0	1	2	3
Facial	Neutral, Smiling	Frown/ grimace	Clenched teeth, full cry	
Body movement	Calm, relaxed	Restless	Moderately agitated	Flailing, agitated
Sleep	Sleeping	Restless when asleep	Intermittent sleep	Unable to sleep, sleep interrupted by jerky movements
Verbal/vocal	No cry	Whimper	Painful crying	Screaming, high-pitched cry when touched
Consolability	Neutral	Easy to console	Not easy to console	Inconsolable
Response to movement/ touch	Moves easily	Winces when touched or moved	Cries when touched or moved	Strong resistance to movement

Three Years and Older

For preschoolers and slightly older, the Faces Pain Rating Scale can be useful. It consists of five faces, the first one with a very happy expression and each of the succeeding ones showing a progressively unhappy expression. The problem with using a face scale (there are others as well, like the Oucher Scale, which uses ten faces) is that you are asking the child to subconsciously integrate into her assessment an element of emotion. There are many reasons why a child may be sad or happy that may not have anything to do with their pain. If a child has just had a fight with his mother, he may feel very sad and so pick a very sad face, but it will not be a clear indication of his level of physical pain.

If a child can count to ten, I ask the child to rate the pain, where 0 is none and 10 is the worst possible imaginable pain. The problem is, if a child's only experience with pain has been a stomachache or skinned knee, he may say the current pain is an 8 or 9 out of 10. But if I ask that question of a child who in the past was hit by a car and then spent time in an intensive care unit, she has a different frame of reference for an 8 or 9 rating. Thus it's easy to see how these tools can result in misleading information.

Naturally, the older a child is, the better she should be able to verbally describe her pain. Again, however, the child's past experiences and frames of reference will influence the description.

RECURRENT ABDOMINAL PAIN (RAP)

"Mommy, my tummy hurts soooo bad."

"I think there's something mean in my stomach. It really, really hurts."

"I don't think I can go to school today. My stomach is killing me."

Most parents have heard these or similar complaints from their children occasionally. But for an estimated 12 percent of girls and 9 percent of boys of preschool and school age, abdominal pain is recurrent or chronic. Recurrent abdominal pain, or RAP, is one of the most common chronic pain complaints that affect children. Among children younger than two years, the cause is usually organic: that is, the pain can be attributed to a biological reason or disease, such as a viral infection, constipation, food allergy, or recurrent urinary tract infection. In older children, however, about 90 percent of cases of recurrent abdominal pain are functional, which means no physical cause can be found. But just because no physical cause can be identified doesn't make the pain any less real. Abdominal pain may be caused by or associated with a disease, such as appendicitis or inflammatory bowel disease (e.g., Crohn's disease, among others), and then treatment of the pain is treatment of the underlying disease itself. But in cases in which abdominal pain is recurrent but *not* associated with any identifiable disease state, a condition I will refer to as RAP, the treatment is more difficult.

Diagnosing RAP

Often we really don't know enough about what's happening in these children to make a definitive diagnosis. That's why I refer to RAP as a "wastebasket" diagnosis, a diagnosis that is made after all structural sources of pain have been excluded. Some children who are given the diagnosis of RAP may eventually—after months or even years of uncertainty by health-care practitioners they visit—be given a diagnosis of irritable bowel syndrome, celiac disease, food allergies, infection with *Helicobacter pylori* (an organism that is responsible for stomach ulcers), or inflammatory bowel disease. A definite diagnosis frequently can't be arrived at quickly because often it's too early in a child's disease course. Therefore when trying to uncover the reason for symptoms of RAP all of these conditions should be considered by your physician and reconsidered periodically over time.

You can help your doctor with the diagnosis of the source of abdominal pain by keeping a pain diary (see Chapter 3) and noting foods, activities, emotional situations, bowel habit changes, and other factors that occur and that may be contributing to or causing your child's pain. You should also keep in mind that children with RAP commonly have other physical symptoms, such as dizziness, headache, and tiredness, and that they are more prone to anxiety and fears than other children their age. Thus when you keep a pain diary, make sure to note other symptoms and emotional reactions your child may experience.

Ultimately, most children who experience severe recurrent abdominal pain must undergo a diagnostic evaluation that rules out the presence of organic diseases, and unfortunately there is no way to do this with a medical history, diary of symptoms, and physical examination alone. X-ray evaluation of the abdomen (often including a computed tomography [CT] scan), as well as a visual inspection and biopsy of the inside of the esophagus, stomach, intestines, and colon by endoscopy are frequently necessary to rule out the presence of a treatable organic problem.

After this kind of extensive evaluation has been done, and if it has proven that there are not any diseases or anatomical abnormalities present at that time, then we are left by the process of elimination with the diagnosis of RAP.

Treatment of RAP and Other Causes of Abdominal Pain

Treatment of abdominal pain depends on its cause. When RAP is characterized by abdominal pain associated with diarrhea, constipation, bloating, gas, and stomach spasms, the diagnosis is probably irritable bowel syndrome (IBS). Because there is not yet a safe and effective medical treatment for this condition, one approach is to teach children how to manage it behaviorally—that is, with self-hypnosis, biofeedback, guided imagery, and relaxation (see Chapter 4). One study at the University of Arizona, for example, found that children who used guided imagery had a 67 percent reduction in pain during therapy. Another approach is physical, as with acupuncture (see Chapter 5). In fact, we've found that acupuncture is very effective in alleviating the pain from IBS in children who stay with the month-long treatment program.

Other organic causes of abdominal pain include celiac disease (an intolerance to gluten, a protein found in wheat flour), or food allergies. If nutritional factors are believed to be behind abdominal pain, then we can make changes to the child's diet until we find the offending food(s) and remove them from the diet. If we have tried behavioral, physical, and nutritional approaches and a child doesn't respond, then we can treat the symptoms. In some cases, I prescribe tricyclic antidepressants, which can help relieve pain as well as improve the quality of sleep at night, or an antiulcer medication such as famotidine (see Chapter 6).

At the same time a child is undergoing any of these treatment approaches, individual and, if needed, family therapy should also be ongoing and considered to be part of the treatment program (see Chapter 7). Why? In the majority of cases of RAP, stress and emotional issues play a large role. One of the main reasons is that children who suffer with RAP typically are highly motivated and highly competitive. Emotional situations at home, at school (which is very often the case), or elsewhere in their environment can affect the severity, frequency, and persistence of their pain. How the children experience and report the pain is amplified and ultimately the parents' response is magnified as well. When everyone's emotions are running high, pain—emotional and physical—is worse. Therefore, individual and/or family counseling with a psychologist or psychiatrist to address the emotional issues is a necessary part of a child's treatment program.

COMPLEX REGIONAL PAIN SYNDROME

At first nothing seemed to be amiss. Twelve-year-old Rebecca appeared to be completely healing and recovering from a sprained ankle that had occurred more than six weeks ago. Then, after coming out of her splint, and without warning, she began to experience swelling all over again, and intense pain in her foot and ankle. X-rays didn't reveal any abnormalities or reason for the pain. Yet the pain was real, very real, and Rebecca, who loved to play soccer, found herself on the sidelines not only for soccer but for just about any walking at all.

Rebecca was diagnosed as having complex regional pain syndrome type 1 (CRPS-1; we will refer to it as CRPS), a condition in which individuals experience pain in one or more limbs and/or the ankles, feet, or hands, that is significantly disproportionate to the original injury and that lingers long after healing of the original trauma has occurred. Generally, CRPS appears after a traumatic event, such as a broken bone, automobile accident, a bad fall, or overuse related to sports. The pain is typically described as burning and sharp, there is coldness and swelling in the affected limb(s), and very typically even light stroking or touching of the skin produces intense feelings of pain, a phenomenon that we call *allodynia*, and one that is characteristic of neuropathic pain syndromes of many sorts.

Complex regional pain syndrome is more common among pre- and adolescent girls than boys by about a 5 to 1 margin, and is usually seen in girls who engage in sports, dancing, or gymnastics. Yet even among this group, it isn't possible to know why if two girls experience the same type of fall, one will develop the condition and the other one will not. This isn't said to frighten you but to let you know that there is no way, as far as we know, you can prevent CRPS. Overuse injuries, trauma, psychological stress, nutritional factors, and hormones have all been named as players in CRPS, yet the actual cause remains unknown.

If left untreated, symptoms of CRPS can become chronic and may even spread to other parts of the body. The unexplained pain can last for years and disrupt childrens' lives by making it difficult or impossible for them to go to school or to participate in after-school activities, sports, and family activities. Children who have CRPS reportedly miss 25 percent of school days.

What Causes Complex Regional Pain Syndrome?

Complex regional pain syndrome is a disease of the autonomic nervous system, which is the system that controls involuntary functions such as blushing, blood pressure, and heart rate. When you are under stress, say, you have to give a speech in front of 100 people, a normal response of the autonomic nervous system might include an increased heart rate, a rise in blood pressure, facial flushing, or sweaty palms. But in people who have CRPS, the autonomic nervous system—specifically a portion of the autonomic nervous system called the sympathetic nervous system—overreacts, but only in certain parts of the body. In CRPS, the part of the body affected is typically one limb, but sometimes more than one. We still don't know exactly why this occurs, but we do have ways to manage and treat it.

Treating CRPS

Children who have CRPS can be treated very effectively, and in most cases drugs are not the first choice. In fact, the primary focus of treatment is physical therapy of the affected body part. But as you might surmise, physical therapy of a painful foot or hand can be itself extremely painful, and most children find themselves unable to tolerate this to any degree. That's where drug therapy and other techniques such as nerve blocks come in handy (see Chapter 6). Children also usually respond very well to mind-body approaches, such as biofeedback, self-hypnosis, acupuncture, relaxation exercises, and hydrotherapy, which we discuss in Chapters 4 and 5 through stories about children who have managed and even eliminated their pain using some of these methods.

Successful treatment of CRPS, in my opinion, also requires psychotherapy for the child and, in many cases, the family as well. Anyone who experiences chronic pain also has emotional issues, such as depression and helplessness, that need to be dealt with, and psychotherapy is instrumental in healing these wounds. Family therapy is often essential because parental response to a child's chronic pain, while given with love and the best intentions, is usually inappropriate and counterproductive. (This statement surprises and even angers some parents, but it is true, as you'll see later.) Thus we find that coaching parents on how to manage and cope with their child's condition helps the child reintegrate into society and strengthens the family unit as well. We discuss these issues in Chapters 7 and 8.

HEADACHE AND MIGRAINE

Chronic, persistent, or recurring head pain from tension-type headache or migraine affects 10 percent of children in the United States. This figure surprises many people, as they tend to think of tension headaches and migraines as being "adult" conditions. Yet we know that by age two years, and in some cases perhaps even earlier, children may experience headache or even migraine. One study suggested that children as young as four months are affected. The researchers arrived at this conclusion when they questioned parents and learned that children at age two years who were having bouts of vomiting doctors believed were associated with headache had also had unexplained vomiting episodes earlier in life. Although the earlier vomiting could not definitely be blamed on headache, it was a viable explanation.

Types of Head Pain

Tension-type headache and migraine are by far the most common types of headache pain experienced by children. Although some parents worry that their child has a brain tumor when chronic headache is the complaint (and one must remember that brain tumors are indeed the most common organ malignancy in children), only about 1,500 children per year have head pain related to a brain tumor. In children, headaches from brain tumors are typically characterized by pain that occurs in the morning, vomiting, loss of coordination, and sometimes seizures. These symptoms can also indicate migraine, so do not jump to conclusions. Your doctor can conduct tests (see "Diagnosis," below) to rule out a brain tumor.

Tension-Type Headache

Tension-type headaches are caused by some type of stressor, physical and/or emotional, that causes constriction of the blood vessels in the head, as well as in other parts of the body, including the shoulders, neck, and face (which can cause facial and jaw pain as well). Eyestrain headache is a type of tension headache in which the child tenses the muscles around the eyes when reading or trying to see the board in school. Fortunately, a quick remedy to this type of tension headache is corrective lenses.

Migraine

When a child is given a diagnosis of migraine, some parents ask, "But isn't my child too young for migraines?" As the study mentioned above suggests, the answer is no. About two thirds of children who have migraines had their first episode by age seven. Boys tend to develop migraines earlier than girls (usually ages six to ten versus ages eleven to fifteen years), but boys also usually outgrow them sooner than girls.

As in adults, symptoms of migraine can vary between children and even between each episode. That's one reason why it's important for you to keep a headache diary and keep careful notes about your child's head pain episodes (see Chapter 3).

Migraines typically are divided into four phases. Your child may or may not experience each of these phases during any given episode.

- Prodrome. This is the period before the head pain actually begins. Not every child experiences this phase. Your child may show some sudden, unusual behaviors, such as unexplained depression or hyperactivity, a craving for a certain food, yawning, restlessness, or excessive thirst. Some children vomit or suddenly get diarrhea or constipation. These symptoms may last a few hours or longer.
- Aura. If this phase occurs at all (only about 5 percent of children with migraine experience aura), it usually happens immediately before the head pain starts, but it can also occur during the headache or even without the headache. The aura phase can be characterized by visual changes, such as seeing flashing lights or colors, black spots, or jagged lines; being oversensitive to light, sound, or touch; vomiting or stomach pain; difficulty speaking; or feeling weak or dizzy. The older your child is, the better he or she will be able to describe any symptoms to you. As you can imagine,

the aura phase can be frightening for children, especially younger ones.

- Headache. In adults, we usually think of migraine as occurring on one side of the head only, but children, especially those younger than twelve years, often say the pain is behind their eyes or in the middle of their forehead. Teenagers are more likely to say that the pain moves from one side of the head to the other, from front to back, or vice versa. The pain can last a few minutes, an hour, or longer, although unlike adults, it rarely lasts more than a day. Note when the headache begins; many times children experience migraine later in the day. Factors that can trigger a migraine include hunger (did your child skip lunch?), dehydration (has your child been playing hard and not drinking fluids?), stress (did your child have a test, confrontation with a classmate, or get a bad report card?), or certain foods (does your child eat chocolate or pepperoni?).
- Resolution. During this phase, the headache may go away suddenly or fade gradually over hours. After a migraine, some children are very tired or depressed, while others feel energetic.

Chronic Daily Headache

Chronic daily headache is head pain that occurs every day or nearly every day for days, weeks, months, or even years. The most common pattern of chronic daily headache in children is a migraine superimposed over frequent tension headaches. This means that the child is caught in a vicious cycle of persistent tension headache with periodic episodes of migraine pain.

Cindy's Story

This was the pattern I saw with Cindy, who was ten years old when she first came to see me with her mother, Jean. There was a strong family history of migraine in the family, and Cindy experienced the classic symptoms: vision disturbances, severe one-sided pain, and fatigue once the episode was over. Along with the periodic migraines, Cindy also had chronic daily headaches which, her mother claimed, were so incapacitating her daughter couldn't go to school several days out of each week, even though she was taking several medications.

As I evaluated Cindy and asked both of them questions about their family and social life, it became clear that Jean doted excessively on her daughter, and Cindy did everything she could to please her mother. Cindy had no close friends, and the fact that she missed so much school didn't help. Jean was a single mother, and she tended to include her daughter in all her plans, leaving Cindy little or no time to socialize with friends her own age.

I made some changes in Cindy's medication and recommended that both Cindy and Jean come into the hospital once a week to talk with a psychologist to help them both better understand Cindy's pain and how to deal with stress and other issues that may be contributing to the headaches. Over the next few months, Cindy and her mother repeatedly missed their appointments with the psychologist and were still unable to manage the headaches at home. At that point I recommended Cindy be hospitalized for a short time so we could try more intensive therapy and medical treatment, but Jean refused because "Cindy doesn't want to stay in any hospital." The migraines and chronic daily headaches continued.

About a month after Jean refused to hospitalize her daughter, Cindy developed trichotillomania—obsessive pulling out of her hair—to the point that she had large bald spots on her head and needed to wear a cap to cover them. Jean finally realized that her daughter desperately needed help, and they both began psychotherapy, with additional group therapy for Cindy. Gradually Jean realized how her desire to keep her daughter close to her was playing a role in Cindy's daily headaches and how Cindy's headache pain, although real, was exaggerated and how she used it to manipulate her mother and avoid going to school.

Cindy's story is an example of how stress and psychological issues can play a key role in a child's chronic pain. We explore this issue in more depth in Chapter 7.

Abdominal Migraine

A variation of the typical migraine is abdominal migraine. The name of this condition often raises eyebrows among parents: How can someone get a migraine in their stomach? The main characteristic of abdominal migraine is repeated, chronic abdominal pain and cyclic vomiting for which there is no apparent cause. The vomiting often lasts for hours and can leave children dehydrated, weak, and fatigued. Some, but not all, children affected with abdominal migraine also experience headache during these episodes. Even when headache is part of the episodes, however, it is often overlooked because of the severity of other symptoms, such as happened with Kathy.

Kathy's Story

For fourteen of her sixteen years, Kathy had been experiencing episodes of recurrent abdominal pain and cyclic vomiting, typically every six to eight weeks. Her mother, Josephine, explained that "Kathy wakes up consistently between ten-thirty and eleven P.M., vomits repeatedly for about twelve hours at least once an hour, then collapses into an exhausted sleep. When she wakes up the next morning, she's tired but doesn't have any pain."

Josephine had taken Kathy to see their pediatrician numerous times over the years, but no cause for the pain or vomiting could be found. "It was frustrating," says Josephine. "No one wants their child to be sick, but I just wanted the doctors to put a name to what was going on. But it seemed like no one could." When Kathy was fifteen years old, her pediatrician referred her to a gastroenterologist, who did extensive testing, including an upper GI, lower GI, CT scan, colonoscopy, and other procedures, and all turned up normal. Tests for allergies also were normal. She was then referred to a neurologist, who prescribed prochlorperazine to stop the vomiting, but it was not effective. He then ordered two different triptans (antimigraine drugs; see Chapter 6) for the same purpose, but although these drugs helped stop the episodes once they started, they did not prevent them. The antianxiety drug alprazolam was also prescribed, and it helped the stomach pain but not the vomiting. At that point, Kathy was referred to my clinic.

The sixteen-year-old girl who walked into my office with her mother was an honor student, star of her high school softball team, and determined to go to college to become a veterinarian. When Kathy, Josephine, and I talked, I asked about stress in Kathy's life, and both she and her mother denied there was anything significant at this time. Josephine felt that her divorce when Kathy was five had likely been stressful, but that the relationship between Kathy and her father was good and had been for many years.

I also learned that Josephine had a history of migraine, although Kathy denied experiencing headaches as part of her symptoms. She did mention, however, that sometimes her episodes were preceded by seeing black spots, tingling in her fingers, thickened saliva, stuffy nose, and paleness. Even though Kathy said she had little or no headache pain, her pre-episode symptoms indicated an aura (see "Migraine"), and that, along with the family history of migraine and her cyclic vomiting, convinced me she had abdominal migraine.

I immediately started Kathy on two treatment approaches: a beta-blocker (nadolol; see Chapter 6) to help prevent migraine; and cognitive-behavioral therapy to help her learn how to manage stress. I continued to follow Kathy closely all through high school, and her episodes of pain and cyclic vomiting steadily decreased to one severe event every five to six months, which she would abort with a triptan. Once she entered college she noticed that her episodes were associated with stress related to final exams, but that other times she felt fine. She asked to be taken off the nadolol, which we did, and she continued to be episode-free for about one year, at which time stress triggered another attack. We decided to put her back on preventive therapy, this time with an antidepressant. She continues to have about one episode per year, and it lasts only a few hours because she treats it with a triptan.

If Kathy's condition had been diagnosed at an earlier age,

she could have been started on specific migraine treatment and probably would have had a more comfortable childhood. However, because she didn't experience any significant headache (but she did have symptoms of aura) and her other symptoms were so severe, the diagnosis was missed. Migraine is a lifetime disorder, and fortunately for Kathy, she has learned ways to manage her stress (progressive relaxation and guided imagery) and has found a medication that keeps the episodes at bay.

Diagnosis

Your child's pediatrician or family practitioner should conduct a thorough examination to evaluate your child's headache. Part of the examination should include a questionnaire in which you, along with your child if he or she is old enough to cooperate, will answer questions about factors such as those listed here. If you've kept a headache diary or any other notes about your child's head pain, you should be well prepared to address these factors:

- associated symptoms such as nausea, vomiting, fatigue, difficulty walking, loss of coordination (such as a change in handwriting), or visual changes
- presence of seizures
- concomitant medical conditions such as sinusitis, high blood pressure, allergies, asthma, or emotional problems
- previous headache history
- what time of day the headache starts, and when it is at its worst
- whether the headaches awaken your child from sleep at night

- whether the headaches prevent your child from normal activities, such as going to school, playing with friends, participating in social events
- what seems to trigger the pain
- what, if anything, seems to relieve the pain
- what, if any, medications does the child take

The doctor should also conduct a thorough neurological exam in which your child's reflexes and nerve responses are checked. This is not a painful or uncomfortable process and involves simple tests like looking at the back of the eyes with a bright light, tapping your child's knee or ankle with a small rubber-tipped instrument, and so on. The doctor may also conduct a CT or magnetic resonance imagery (MRI) scan to rule out an anatomical cause, such as a brain tumor, for the pain if there are any abnormalities in the physical examination, or any suspicious features in the history of the headaches.

Treatment

Treatment of tension headache, migraine, or chronic daily headache depends on the frequency and severity of the pain. In children who experience infrequent head pain, say, once a month or less, I prefer to treat each incidence of headache rather than prescribing daily medication to prevent headache. These medications to relieve head pain can be helpful, but only in the short term.

What can be even more effective and longer lasting—and without the risk of side effects—are cognitive-behavioral therapies, such as biofeedback, self-hypnosis, relaxation exercises, and visualization. In a study of teenagers who had migraine, for example, researchers found that cognitive-behavioral therapies worked better than triptan drugs.

But if headache or migraine is occurring more frequently than once a month, or if a child has chronic daily headache, I usually recommend a combination of a preventive approach, using medications, cognitive-behavioral therapies to reduce stress (see Chapter 4), as well as physical therapies such as acupuncture and exercise (see Chapter 5), in addition to medication to treat each headache as it occurs. It is very important to address any psychological and emotional issues that are compounding chronic headache, and so I encourage parents and children to participate in some individual and/or family therapy sessions (see Chapter 7).

Drugs are prescribed as needed. Most children, even those with migraine headaches, respond well to occasional use of over-the-counter nonsteroidal antiinflammatory drugs such as ibuprofen (Advil, Motrin, etc.). Although not approved by the FDA for use in children, the class of drugs known as triptans has proven very useful in treating episodic childhood migraine that doesn't respond to over-the-counter medication. These drugs include sumatriptan (Imitrex), frovatriptan (Frova), rizatriptan (Maxalt), and zolmitriptan (Zomig). The risks and benefits of acetaminophen, ibuprofen, aspirin, triptans, and other drugs, all of which can be used for head pain, are discussed in Chapter 6. A new and effective treatment of both migraine and chronic daily headache is the injection of botulinum toxin A (Botox) or B (Myobloc), a therapeutic form of the toxin produced by the germ that causes botulism poisoning, and is also discussed in Chapter 6.

FIBROMYALGIA SYNDROME (FMS)

Fibromyalgia is a chronic condition in which individuals experience widespread pain in their muscles and in the areas around the joints, especially where the muscles attach to the bone, as well as moderate to severe fatigue. In children and adolescents, the condition is called juvenile primary fibromyalgia. One reason we distinguish between adult and childhood fibromyalgia is that although the symptoms are similar, the outcome is usually better for young people than adults.

Studies differ as to how common this condition is among children: one study found that 1.2 percent of school-age children—all females—met the criteria for the disease, while others have found a higher prevalence. In fact, juvenile primary fibromyalgia is seen almost exclusively in girls. The disease typically develops after age thirteen and is most commonly diagnosed at fifteen.

Many of the individuals affected are like Tabitha, a fifteen-year-old who was frustrated not only with her symptoms but with her doctors and her parents. Before Tabitha was referred to my hospital, her parents had taken her to two other doctors, who had not come up with a diagnosis. When I examined her, I recognized the symptoms of fibromyalgia: very painful trigger points (specific areas on the body known to correspond to fibromyalgia when pressure is applied to them), fatigue, and headache. Tabitha also reported sleep difficulties, and she was both anxious and depressed.

Tabitha was a good student and had been active in various activities, including the school drama club, the swim team, and the school orchestra, where she played the flute. For the past four months, however, she had found it increasingly impossible to keep up with school work, and she had had to drop out of the swim team because of fatigue and muscle pain. Some days she would go to school, only to be extremely fatigued by midmorning. Her anxiety about missing school and feeling "like a freak" because she often was too exhausted to go out with her friends was causing her to be depressed.

Cause and Diagnosis

The cause of fibromyalgia is unknown. Some researchers believe there may be a link with psychological stress, immune or hormone abnormalities, or sleep disturbance. More recently, evidence points to lower than normal levels of endogenous (naturally produced) opioids in the central nervous system, such as endorphins, as the cause of FMS. This finding makes a lot of sense, when one sees the unusual and enhanced amount of pain that girls with FMS have all over their body in response to pressure that ordinarily would not cause pain in other children.

Several studies suggest that genetics play at least some role in the disease. In one study, 28 percent of the children of mothers who had fibromyalgia also developed the disease. In another, 66 percent of parents of children who had juvenile primary fibromyalgia had chronic pain, and about 10 percent of them had fibromyalgia. It's also been shown that families who are very close emotionally are more likely to have severe cases of juvenile primary fibromyalgia.

Many pediatricians are not familiar with fibromyalgia and may overlook the diagnosis, as was the case with Tabitha's previous two doctors. Missing the diagnosis is not uncommon, especially as symptoms of the disease are similar to those of other medical conditions. Indeed, fibromyalgia can be a challenge to identify, as there are no laboratory tests that can confirm a diagnosis. Your doctor may use X-rays and other tests, however, to rule out other causes of the symptoms, most importantly diseases such as lupus erythematosus or rheumatoid arthritis, but it should be remembered that a diagnosis of fibromyalgia is not just a process of elimination. There are criteria for its diagnosis. In order to have a diagnosis of FMS, one must have at least eighteen pressure points at typical areas in the body that produce unusual degrees of pain, as well as associated symptoms of fatigue and headache.

Treatment

Thus far we don't have a cure for fibromyalgia, and I had to relay this fact to Tabitha, as I do to the other young people who have this condition. However, there are some positive aspects to fibromyalgia, and one is that there are many effective therapies and medications from which to choose. Another good thing about fibromyalgia is that although it is painful and can be debilitating at times, it does not cause physical damage to the tissues. Thus, treatment should always include physical therapy and a regular aerobic exercise program. And depending on your child's overall health, medical history, severity of symptoms, and tolerance and acceptance of different therapies, heat and/or cold treatments, massage, relaxation and stress management techniques, and, if needed, medications can be introduced (see Chapters 4, 5, and 6).

In Tabitha's case, I encouraged her to return to swimming,

not on a competitive level but as a way to maintain flexibility, strength, and conditioning. Although she often experienced fatigue, I emphasized that mild, regular exercise in a pool would be an excellent part of her therapy. Tabitha also worked with a physical therapist once a week who monitored her exercise program and made sure she stayed on track, and she also agreed to attend biofeedback sessions, where she learned to control her pain.

It's important not to overlook the psychological factors when treating juvenile primary fibromyalgia, and so I urged Tabitha's parents to take her to a child psychologist. A recent study (October 2003) in *Arthritis and Rheumatology* reported that children with this syndrome have increased levels of anxiety and depression, higher pain sensitivity, more temperamental instability, and less family cohesion than healthy children or children who have arthritis. The parents of these children also reported higher levels of depression and anxiety and less ability to cope when compared with parents of the other two groups. Thus individual and often family therapy is an essential part of the treatment program for children who have juvenile primary fibromyalgia (see Chapter 7).

ARTHRITIS

There are several forms of arthritis that afflict children, and none of them are good. Juvenile rheumatoid arthritis (JRA) is the most common, but children also may contract systemic lupus erythematosus (SLE, or lupus), or ankylosing spondylitis, for example. Because JRA is the most common form of arthritis in children, and because the pain and the management of the pain are very similar for each of these causes, I'll limit my discussion to JRA.

When parents are told their child has juvenile rheumatoid arthritis, some think it's a big mistake. Although rheumatoid arthritis is a disease that is much more common among older people, a juvenile form affects 70,000 to 100,000 children in the United States. Juvenile rheumatoid arthritis is the most common rheumatic disease that affects children, and is defined as arthritis that causes stiffness and joint inflammation for more than six weeks in a child who is sixteen years or younger. This disease is classified into three types, based on certain factors:

- Pauciarticular. This is the most common form of juvenile rheumatoid arthritis. It is seen in about 50 percent of children who have the disease. The disease typically appears in children around age three years, although it can appear in children as young as one year. It is also much more likely to develop in girls. In pauciarticular JRA, four or fewer joints are affected, with large joints (e.g., knees) usually falling victim. The majority of children who have pauciarticular JRA have only one joint affected, usually the knee. Some children have certain antibodies in their blood, including the antinuclear antibody (ANA) and rheumatoid factor (RF). Approximately 20 to 30 percent of children with pauciarticular JRA also have eye disease, and up to 80 percent of them also have ANA in their blood. For children with this combination of factors, JRA usually develops at an earlier age. Pauciarticular JRA disappears in some children as they reach adulthood, but eye problems can persist, and in some people joint symptoms recur.

- Polyarticular. In polyarticular JRA (which affects about 30 percent of all children with JRA), five or more joints are affected. Joints in the feet and hands are most often involved, but larger joints may also be affected. Children with polyarticular JRA who also have an antibody in their blood called IgM rheumatoid factor (RF) are usually more seriously affected than children who do not. This is the form of JRA that most closely resembles rheumatoid arthritis in adults.
- Systemic. The systemic form of JRA causes fever and rash, along with joint swelling, and may also affect various organs, such as the heart, spleen, and liver. About 20 percent of children with JRA get this form of the disease. The antibodies ANA and RF are rarely seen in these children.

Regardless of the type of JRA, the most common symptoms are persistent joint swelling, pain, and stiffness that is usually worse after a nap or a night's sleep. The first indication of JRA some parents have is that their child begins to limp, especially in the morning when he or she first gets up. Although children may have pain and limited movement in an affected joint, they may not complain.

Cause and Diagnosis

Juvenile rheumatoid arthritis, like the form that develops in adults, is an autoimmune disease, which means the body perceives some of its own cells as "the enemy" and attacks them with antibodies and white blood cells. This attack on healthy tissue causes inflammation, redness, heat and, of course, pain. No one has yet discovered why the body initiates these attacks, although some experts believe it is a combination of genetics and an environmental trigger, such as a virus or toxin.

No single test can definitely identify JRA. Thus your doctor will take note of your child's symptoms (including any observations you have made; here's where keeping a pain diary will be very helpful) and gather information from various tests, including complete blood count, urinalysis, liver function tests, kidney function tests, erythrocyte sedimentation rate (ESR; a high rate on this test indicates inflammation in the body), and several blood tests that detect antibodies in the blood.

One thing the doctor will look for in the blood count is a positive rheumatoid factor (RF). Rheumatoid factor is an example of an autoantibody. (An antibody is a type of protein that destroys bacteria and other foreign materials in the body; an autoantibody reacts with a person's own cells.) The presence of RF is not a "sure sign" that a person has JRA, as it can be found in people who have other types of inflammatory conditions as well. However, it is important for your doctor to check for RF because children with JRA who have this autoantibody tend to have a more aggressive and persistent form of JRA. Fortunately, only about 5 percent of children with polyarticular JRA have a positive RF test. These children are at higher risk of developing permanent joint damage and may have arthritis that lasts into adulthood. Therefore, doctors usually recommend more aggressive treatment for these patients.

About 95 percent of children with polyarticular JRA have

a negative RF blood test. These children generally experience a few years of ups and downs with the disease—episodes of flare-ups followed by remission—after which the symptoms fade away.

Another type of autoantibody your doctor will look for in the blood test is antinuclear antibodies, or ANAs. Like rheumatoid factors, ANAs can be found in people who don't have rheumatic conditions. Between 40 and 60 percent of children with JRA have a positive ANA test, and most of these children have pauciarticular JRA. The presence of ANA is important because it places a child at higher risk of developing iritis, inflammation of the iris in the eye.

Course of the Disease

Children who have JRA (as well as the other forms of arthritis) can experience a rollercoaster of symptoms: some days or weeks may be nearly pain free while other days or weeks may not. Pain may be worse in the morning, then subside later in the day. Every child's experience with JRA is different, so you will want to take note of factors that seem to trigger your child's pain as well as things that seem to relieve it.

Because children who have the pauciarticular form of JRA (and several other forms of childhood autoimmune arthritis and bowel diseases) are susceptible to some eye diseases, such as iritis and uveitis (inflammation of the uvea), they should be examined by an ophthalmologist every three to four months. Symptoms of these eye disorders often don't develop until the symptoms of JRA have been apparent for some time, so it's important to have an eye examination as soon as JRA has been diagnosed. If iritis is not identified and treated early, permanent vision loss may result.

Another concern is growth problems, which can affect some children, depending on the severity of the disease and the joints involved. Some children experience a slowing of growth overall, while others find that one leg or arm grows faster than the other, especially among children who have pauciarticular JRA. Generally, the limb affected by arthritis grows faster than the unaffected limb because there is an increased supply of blood in the arthritic limb. This size discrepancy can be upsetting to children, but it's important to let them know that the difference will disappear once the inflammation subsides. Children who have one leg shorter than the other may need to wear a shoe lift until the legs even out.

Treatment

When we treat a child who has painful JRA or another form of arthritis, after working with our colleagues in the specialty of rheumatology to be sure the medical management of the arthritis has been optimized, our primary concern is to help our patient have the best value of life possible. That means we work to reduce swelling and pain, maintain as much movement as possible, and prevent any complications. Thus we turn to physical therapists and occupational therapists, who can show you how to do simple exercises with your child at home, as well as massage (see Chapter 5). We also consider which medications are most appropriate, including nonsteroidal antiinflammatory drugs (NSAIDs), disease-modifying antirheumatic drugs (DMARDs), and corticosteroids (see Chapter 6). Complementary approaches, including acupuncture, biofeedback, hydrotherapy, self-hypnosis, and visualization/guided imagery have also proven helpful (see Chapters 4 and 5).

ENDOMETRIOSIS

"My daughter can't have endometriosis," said Eileen, whose fourteen-year-old daughter Janelle was suffering with severe abdominal and pelvic pain. "She's too young, isn't she?"

Eileen's question is not uncommon; most people associate endometriosis, a disease that affects females in their reproductive years, with women in their twenties and thirties, not teenage girls. The Endometriosis Association notes that endometriosis affects an estimated 5.5 million women and adolescent girls in the United States. The exact number of teenage girls who are affected is not known, but I believe the condition is greatly underdiagnosed in this age group. Some experts believe that endometriosis is responsible for 45 to 70 percent of chronic abdominal or pelvic pain in teenage girls.

What Is Endometriosis?

Endometriosis is a hormonal and immune condition that involves the endometrium, the tissue that lines the inside of the uterus and which builds up and sheds each month during a female's menstrual cycle. In some females, however, the endometrium also grows outside the uterus and forms growths, sometimes referred to as nodules, tumors, or lesions. These growths can appear on the outside of the uterus on the ovaries, fallopian tubes, lining of the pelvic or abdominal cavity, ligaments that support the uterus, and in the area around the rectum and vagina.

The endometrium responds to the release of hormones during the menstrual cycle. For the endometrium inside the uterus, this means that it is shed in menstrual blood. The endometrium in other parts of the body, however, has no place to go, and causes internal bleeding, inflammation, and the formation of scar tissue. The bottom line is, endometriosis is painful. It can cause severe menstrual cramps (before and during periods), pain in the middle of the menstrual cycle when the endometrium is becoming engorged, lower back pain, painful bowel movements, diarrhea, constipation, and fatigue.

Causes

Although no one is sure what causes endometriosis, there are several theories. One is that some of the endometrium makes its way up through the fallopian tubes, gets into the abdomen, and grows there. Another is that endometrial tissue is transported in the blood or lymph to other parts of the body. Some research shows that environmental toxins such as dioxin, which acts like hormones in the body, cause endometriosis in animals and may do the same thing in humans. Finally, there seems to be a genetic component, because it is more common in girls whose mothers have had endometriosis.

Diagnosis

Although a doctor may sometimes feel growths during a pelvic examination, the only way to arrive at a definite diagnosis is to perform a laparoscopy and look around the pelvic and abdominal spaces. A laparoscopy is a surgical procedure in which a small tube (laparoscope) with a light in it is inserted into a tiny incision that is made in the abdomen. The surgeon can then examine the area around the abdomen for endometrial growths.

For many young women, finding a doctor who recognizes the symptoms of endometriosis and accepts the fact that this condition occurs in adolescents is a challenge. I have known patients who have gone from doctor to doctor and were told they were probably suffering with gastrointestinal problems or even that their pain was "in their head." Some were told outright that they were "too young" to have endometriosis. Persistence, and finding the right doctor, one experienced in the gynecology of adolescents, and most importantly one who is an expert at laparoscopy, are the keys to an accurate diagnosis (see Chapter 3, Finding Professional Help).

I am reminded of Stephanie, a tall, athletic young lady of fifteen who was experiencing severe pelvic pain during her menstrual cycle. Before she came to our center, she had fortunately found a gynecologist who suspected endometriosis and ordered a laparoscopy. But the results were normal, so she suggested Stephanie was, for some reason, exaggerating the severity of her symptoms. "Girls get cramps," she said to her mother. "Give her ibuprofen and she'll be fine."

But her pain got worse and worse, and she had to abandon her athletic activities because running and jumping brought on incapacitating pain in her abdomen. When Stephanie was brought to see me by her mother and I reviewed the case, I completely disagreed with the doctor's assessment. Not only had

Stephanie given up her position as star center on her school's basketball team, she had also reached a point where it was too painful for her to sit in a moving car on a bumpy road. This young lady was not faking or exaggerating her pain. I noted that the laparoscopy had been done when Stephanie had been in the least pain, but I believed a more accurate picture of what was happening would be seen if the test was done when she was in greatest pain. I recommended she undergo another laparoscopy by a surgeon whom I knew to be an expert laparoscopist, and the results showed a large endometrial growth on one of her ovaries. The growth was removed surgically, and since then she has had no pain.

Treatment

Not every case of endometriosis ends in the operating room; in fact, many do not. I have found that acupuncture is very effective in treating the pain associated with this condition, as are exercise and hydrotherapy (see Chapter 5). These can be used along with antiinflammatory drugs, such as ibuprofen (see Chapter 6) and relaxation techniques (see Chapter 4). Also, many girls respond well to low-dose birth control pills, which prevent the endometrial tissues from becoming engorged and painful.

Addressing the emotional needs of adolescents who have endometriosis is also vitally important. Severe cramps and sleep deprivation often keep girls out of school for days or even weeks before and during their period. Family members, teachers, and friends may wonder what's so bad about "some cramps" and girls are often told that "cramps are normal, so live with them." Teenagers who suffer with endometriosis can be made to feel inferior, weird, or wimpy. These girls often cannot participate in normal teenage activities, both at school and during leisure time. Thus psychological support, including individual therapy and support groups, is encouraged as part of the treatment plan (see Chapter 7).

CANCER PAIN

It's been said that the words "cancer" and "children" should never appear in the same sentence. Unfortunately, cancer strikes 1 out of every 330 children in the United States—in 1999, approximately 20,000 children and adolescents were diagnosed with some form of the disease. And many of these children experience chronic, persistent pain.

One thing that always surprises me is that many oncologists wait so long to refer a pediatric cancer patient to a pain management specialist. The sooner these children can participate in a specialized pain management program, the less they will suffer. Sometimes the factor that drives oncologists to wait so long is an exaggerated idea, among both doctors and the public, of a risk of addiction to opioids. We will talk more about this misconception later in Chapter 6, but for now know that addiction to opioids (given for cancer pain) among children is rare, while the relief they can provide a child who is suffering is priceless.

Causes of Cancer-Related Pain

The pain associated with cancer can come from both the disease and the treatment. Tumors can cause severe pain from many different reasons, including bone pain, neuropathic (nerve) pain, or stretching of membranes around cancerous organs, depending on their size, location, and other factors. Chemotherapy—the use of drugs to attack the cancer—often is accompanied by even more challenges, such as nausea, vomiting, fatigue, ulceration of the mouth, and painful neuropathies (pain caused by damage to the nerves). Many of the procedures related to cancer treatment are also painful, including lumbar punctures (also known as spinal taps, when a needle is used to withdraw cerebrospinal fluid from the spinal column), collection of bone marrow samples, surgical procedures to remove tumors, and even the repeated taking of blood samples. We talk about how to deal with these types of painful procedures as well in Part II.

Treatment

Treatment of cancer is typically multifaceted, highly individualized, and can include anticancer therapy, such as chemotherapy, surgery, and radiotherapy; for treatment of cancer-related pain, mind-body techniques such as meditation, guided imagery, self-hypnosis, biofeedback, and relaxation therapy are useful in addition to painkillers and nerve blocks. These approaches are discussed in Part II of this book.

The goal is always to improve a child's comfort and function, without sacrificing function for comfort except at the end of life. Sometimes a child is given, say, an opioid on a regular dosing schedule, but he or she experiences breakthrough pain—pain that occurs before the next scheduled dose of medication. If the doctor does not prescribe a medication for the breakthrough pain, the child is undermedicated and is not being offered the chance to function as fully as possible. However, if a child is medicated to the point that he or she can't get out of bed or interact with family and friends, then the child is overmedicated. In both cases the pain management program needs to be reevaluated. Bringing in a pain management specialist early in the course of the disease can help prevent avoidable pain and overmedication (see Chapter 3).

The type and degree of treatment also depend on whether we are treating recoverable or terminal cancer. In children who have recoverable cancer, it is best to minimize the use of drugs, especially opioids, not because there is a risk of addiction (remember, addiction to these drugs is virtually nonexistent among children), but because children pay a price in the form of side effects for taking these drugs: constipation, sweating, loss of appetite, nausea, vomiting, dizziness, and drowsiness. Plus, when opioids are used for a lengthy period of time, drug tolerance may develop, which means that larger and larger doses are needed to maintain effectiveness, and that over time the drug may become less and less effective. This would limit our ability to treat escalating pain later in the course of the disease, if things worsen. In addition, prolonged and continuous use of opioids leads to physical dependence; while this is not the same thing as addiction, physical dependence may be a problem because if the opioid is abruptly decreased in dose or discontinued, then very unpleasant symptoms of withdrawal will occur. Thus, doctors should try to incorporate as many nondrug treatments as the child and parents are able or willing to try and that prove to be effective, along with appropriate drug use.

In children who have terminal cancer, doctors can be more aggressive with the use of opioids. That's not to say that other approaches should not be tried; they should, and we have had success with visualization, biofeedback, and self-hypnosis in children who are terminally ill with cancer.

OTHER CHRONIC PAIN CONDITIONS

We have grouped several other painful childhood conditions together, not because they are less important—all conditions that cause childhood pain are important—but because they are less prevalent. Although we have given less space to background information on these conditions, you are referred to more complete coverage on treatment options in Part II.

Back Pain

Thankfully, chronic back pain among children is not nearly as common as it is among adults; however, 5 percent of children do experience some type of persistent problem. Here are some of the more common causes.

Spondylolysis. Research indicates that by age six years, 4.4 percent of children are already affected by spondylolysis, a painful condition caused by a defect in the lower vertebrae of the spinal column. Possible causes of spondylolysis include an inherited tendency for the vertebral bone to be thin; or overuse, especially participation in sports such as gymnastics, weight lifting, and football, which may cause a stress fracture in the lower back. The pain is usually worse when children are active and improves when they rest. In fact, treatment for spondylolysis, in most cases, includes rest, use of nonsteroidal antiinflammatory drugs (see Chapter 6), and stretching and strengthening exercises, which can be facilitated by a physical therapist and then continued at home. In mild cases, children can usually participate in activities that spare the back from too much stress, such as swimming or walking. More severe cases may require that the child wear a back brace or even corrective orthopedic surgery to stabilize the spine.

Diskitis. An infection that affects the space between the disks in the back can also cause chronic back pain in children. Called diskitis, it also causes fever and muscle spasms in the back. Some children are so uncomfortable they refuse to stand or walk. Diskitis can be diagnosed using a bone scan or magnetic resonance imaging (MRI), which can detect whether the infection has caused the disk space to become narrow. Treatment involves bed rest and, in some cases, use of antibiotics (see Chapter 6).

Sports Injuries. The most common cause of acute back pain in children is sports injuries. Fortunately, the majority of these incidents involve only a strain or a pulled muscle, and treatment with nonsteroidal antiinflammatory drugs like ibuprofen (see Chapter 6), along with an ice pack and some rest, allows the pain to go away in five to seven days, and chronic pain is not a problem. If the pain should continue beyond seven days, you should see a doctor for an evaluation.

Facial Pain

It's been estimated that chronic facial pain affects about 5 percent of children in the United States. The main culprits are ear infections, sinusitis, and temporomandibular joint disorder (TMD).

Ear Infections. Middle ear infections are very common in children. In fact, about two-thirds of children younger than three years old experience at least one acute middle ear infection episode, which typically lasts up to two weeks. Some of these acute infections, however, progress to chronic cases, characterized by continuous or intermittent ear pain, feeling of fullness in the ear, pus-like drainage from the ear, and loss of hearing. In children who are too young to tell parents how they feel, other telltale indications are pulling on the ear, irritability, and difficulty eating and sleeping.

Treatment of chronic ear infections may take several months of dosing with antibiotics (if the infection is bacterial) in oral form or ear drops. Hot or cold compresses held on the ear can also help the pain. Sometimes surgical removal of the adenoids is necessary to allow the Eustachian tube (the passageway that leads from the back of the throat to the ear) to open.

Sinusitis. Sinusitis—infection and inflammation of the sinus cavities—is a common chronic disease among children. One reason children are prone to sinusitis is that their sinus cavities are still developing during childhood and do not reach maturity until around age twenty.

Because symptoms of sinusitis and a cold are similar, it's important to note how long your child has symptoms of a cold. Those symptoms generally include headache, runny nose with discharge of thick yellow or greenish mucus, stuffy nose, low fever, tenderness around the nose and below the eyes, tiredness, weakness, and cough that may be worse at night. If the symptoms last for more than ten days, your child probably has acute sinusitis. If the symptoms persist for more than a few months, the diagnosis may be chronic sinusitis.

The most common treatment for chronic sinusitis is antibiotics to fight infection and decongestants to reduce the swelling inside of the nose and sinuses to permit proper drainage. If, however, allergy is causing inflammation, an antihistamine may be prescribed. Oral and/or nasal steroids are also used in some cases (see Chapter 6). Treatment of chronic sinusitis may take up to six weeks or longer, and occasionally surgery is necessary to get out all the infection and to permit the sinuses to drain.

Temporomandibular Joint Disorder. Pain and discomfort in the jaw muscles and jaw joints (temporomandibular, or TM joints) is called temporomandibular disorder (TMD). These joints, which are in front of each ear and connect the lower jawbone to the skull, are flexible and move when people talk, swallow, chew, smile, and so on. Thus children with TMD can experience pain on one or both sides of the jaw, as well as painful grating sensations or clicking, when they open their mouth to talk, chew, or yawn. Other symptoms of TMD include headache, an inability to open the jaw wide, and locking of the jaw in an open or closed position.

The most common cause of temporomandibular disorder is tension in the muscles that control the jaw, such as tension caused when children clench their jaw or grind their teeth. Tension in the jaw can also be caused by myofascial pain dysfunction syndrome, which is pain in the tissues that surround the jaw muscles, as well as injury to the jaw or face, arthritis in the joint, or a structural problem present at birth. Treatment typically includes rest, antiinflammatory drugs, and physical therapy.

Sickle Cell Anemia

Sickle cell anemia is an inherited blood condition that affects about 72,000 people in the United States, most of whom can trace their ancestry to Africa. Hispanic-Americans are also affected, but rarely so.

In sickle cell anemia, the structure of the hemoglobin (the substance in red blood cells that carries oxygen) is abnormal, causing the red blood cells themselves to become irregularly shaped, like a sickle. This unusual shape causes the red blood cells to clump together. Then they get trapped in tiny spaces in the bone, causing severe bone pain. When the cells gather in small blood vessels throughout the body, they can reduce or eliminate blood flow to certain areas, including organs. When this occurs, it is known as a *sickle cell crisis* and it is often preceded by and caused by an infection accompanied by a fever and possibly dehydration.

Crises are very painful and can last hours or days. They also can cause serious damage to the organ that is affected. Blocked flow to the brain, for example, can cause paralysis or stroke, while reduced blood to the kidneys can cause kidney failure. Therefore it is critically important for parents to seek immediate medical attention if their child experiences sudden pain in any part of the body or develops an infection. Prompt treatment of an infection can help prevent a crisis from occurring. If one does occur, children need to begin taking pain-killing drugs immediately and to drink lots of fluids to rehydrate their blood and help keep their blood flowing as freely as possible. If the pain is severe, morphine or other opioids may be given, while antibiotics may be necessary to fight infection. Some children need to be hospitalized during their crisis; others may be sent home with medication and instructions to continue to drink lots of fluids.

Because an infection can be deadly in children who have sickle cell anemia, doctors typically start infants as young as two months of age on a daily routine of oral penicillin until they are about five years old. This is done to help prevent pneumococcal infection, which can cause early death.

Depending on the age of the child, various mind-body therapies can be helpful in relieving pain, including self-hypnosis, biofeedback, progressive relaxation, and guided imagery/visualization, which also help children develop self-esteem and reduce stress (see Chapter 4). Acupuncture and TENS (transcutaneous electrical nerve stimulation) have also proved helpful for some patients. Exercise, including participation in sports, is encouraged as much as the child is able to handle safely.

Unlike some conditions that involve chronic pain, sickle cell anemia is a lifelong, sometimes fatal disease. Thus emotional support and guidance from support groups, as well as a psychologist, are especially critical for both the child and the family (see Chapters 3 and 7, respectively).

Irritable Bowel Syndrome

Irritable bowel syndrome is a digestive disorder in which the intestinal muscles don't contract properly, or in coordination.

The result is that digested food moves through the intestines either too fast, which causes gas, bloating, and diarrhea; or too slowly, causing constipation, bloating, and cramps. In children we see two types of irritable syndrome: diarrhea-dominant disease, which occurs in children younger than five years old; and pain-dominant disease, seen in children older than five.

Diarrhea-dominant irritable bowel syndrome is usually painless and may include periodic bouts of constipation. In pain-dominant disease, the pain typically occurs around the navel in younger children and usually in the lower left abdomen in older children. Other symptoms of irritable bowel syndrome may include headache, mucus in the stool, weight loss (in children who eat less because of the pain), and nausea.

Stress can trigger symptoms of irritable bowel syndrome, but it does not cause the disease. Other triggers include eating gas-producing foods, such as fatty or fried foods, chocolate, carbonated beverages, beans, and raw vegetables. Another condition that may mimic irritable bowel syndrome is lactose intolerance, which means the body cannot digest lactose, a sugar in dairy products.

Irritable bowel syndrome is sometimes identified as the cause of recurrent abdominal pain (see "Recurrent Abdominal Pain" in this chapter). Diagnosis of irritable bowel syndrome depends on the child's history and the doctor's findings when she examines the child. Doctors look for signs of infection and inflammation, and to accomplish that they take blood tests, a urinalysis, stool samples, abdominal X-ray, and lactose breath hydrogen test (to test for lactose intolerance). In some cases, a colonoscopy is ordered as well. The good news is that irritable bowel syndrome doesn't cause damage to the intestines. Like the case for fibromyalgia syndrome, there are specific criteria for diagnosing irritable bowel syndrome in adults (for example, the Rome Criteria, which were developed during an international conference of experts in Rome several years ago), but their applicability to children is unknown. Very much like migraine headaches, the well-defined symptoms of IBS in adults may not occur as typically in children. The bottom line is that recurrent chronic abdominal pain in children that is associated with gas, changes in bowel habits, or mucus in the stools is probably irritable bowel syndrome, provided, of course, that other organic causes of abdominal pain have been ruled out.

Treatment of irritable bowel syndrome typically includes stress management techniques, such as biofeedback, self-hypnosis, progressive relaxation, and visualization/guided imagery, as well as dietary changes, including the addition of more fiber to the child's diet and the elimination of some fat. Acetaminophen may also be prescribed. Laxatives and antidiarrheal medications are usually not recommended unless the symptoms cannot be controlled using stress management and diet, because the body can become dependent on them. Opioids are never of any benefit because they themselves will lead to constipation and abdominal pain, as well as physical dependence and tolerance.

HIV/AIDS

According to the Centers for Disease Control and Prevention, more than 45,000 people age twenty-four years and younger in the United States have human immunodeficiency virus (HIV). Several studies conducted in children with HIV show that more than half of them experience significant pain, including neuromuscular pain, abdominal pain, headache, chest pain, pain while swallowing, muscle pain, earache, and mouth pain.

Treatment of pain in children with HIV can range from mild analgesics such as nonsteroidal antiinflammatory drugs to antiseizure drugs, antidepressants, and opioids (see Chapter 6). If the pain is severe, doctors may prescribe more than one opioid—one long-lasting drug for basic relief and one short-acting opioid for breakthrough pain.

Nonpharmaceutical approaches to HIV pain in children include acupuncture, visualization/guided imagery, meditation, self-hypnosis, and progressive relaxation.

Cystic Fibrosis

Approximately 30,000 children and adults in the United States have cystic fibrosis, the most common genetic disease in the United States, in which the body produces abnormally thick mucus that obstructs the lungs and pancreas, which makes it difficult to breathe, results in frequent and severe respiratory infections, and impairs the ability of the body to digest food. These repeated infections eventually lead to permanent lung damage. In addition to wheezing and shortness of breath, other symptoms of cystic fibrosis include persistent coughing, frequent respiratory infections, and excessive appetite but poor weight gain. Since many different organs can be affected by cystic fibrosis, pain can occur in many parts of the body and result in abdominal pain, sinusitis, headache, and muscle pain.

Treatment includes use of antibiotics for each episode of respiratory infection, nonsteroidal antiinflammatory drugs (although these are used cautiously because of their association with bleeding problems, plus their ability to promote asthma attacks), plus daily physical therapy to help drain mucus from the lungs. Some studies have found that acupuncture, massage, and meditation are also helpful for some patients (see Chapters 4 and 5). At the end of life for patients with cystic fibrosis, opioids are used to treat chest pain and reduce the sensation of not getting enough air to breathe, which is called air hunger.

BOTTOM LINE

One of the most important tools you as parents can have to help your child who lives with chronic pain is an understanding of the cause of that pain. While knowledge doesn't make the physical pain disappear, it can relieve some of the anxiety, frustration, and fear you and your child may be living with every day. The information presented in this chapter is a launching point for you to explore further: to ask questions of your health-care practitioners, read the literature, search the Internet, and talk with other parents and children who share your situation and concerns. When we all work together, we can learn even more about how to bring relief to the millions of children who suffer with chronic or persistent pain.

Part II

A Program to Treat Your Child's Chronic Pain

Chapter 3

FINDING PROFESSIONAL HELP

As a parent who has a child living with chronic pain, one of your priorities is to find experienced, knowledgeable, and compassionate medical professionals whom you can count on to help you and your child cope with and manage the pain and to improve your child's quality of life. When you know you can count on such individuals, much of the stress, fear, and anxiety that can be associated with helping a child who has chronic pain can be alleviated. Similarly, when you and your child have assistance from outside the medical circle, such as from support groups and concerned individuals, feelings of frustration and alienation can disappear. What kind of professionals do you need to contact? Where can you find them? How do you know if they are the right ones for your child's needs?

Children can't find their own medical professional help, so that task is up to you, their parents. Finding the most appropriate team can be a challenge, but in this chapter we take the angst out of the search by explaining how to find a pediatrician who specializes in pain, how to find a pain management clinic, and the benefits of working with a team of professionals (pediatricians, psychologists, physical therapists) at such clinics. We also talk about how to create and use a pain diary, which you may find invaluable when interacting with your child's pain management team, and about the benefits of joining both live and online support groups.

GETTING A DIAGNOSIS

We are going to assume that you are just beginning your search for the reason behind your child's pain. Naturally, if you already have a diagnosis, you may wish to move ahead to a more appropriate section, such as "Finding a Qualified Pediatric Pain Practitioner" or "Working with a Pain Management Team." However, you may want to read through this section if you've been thinking about changing your child's doctor or you want to make sure you've explored all your options before making a choice.

Your Insurance

In this age of managed health care, many people are limited in their options when it comes to choosing which doctors and hospitals they can go to, unless, of course, they choose to seek medical care outside their insurance plan and pay a large co-payment or even entirely out-of-pocket. Depending on your plan, you may have significant, little, or no choice as to which doctor you can see. Therefore, your first step is to review your plan or speak with your plan's manager to find out what your options are:

- How many pediatricians are on the list from which you can choose a doctor?

- What happens if you don't like the doctor you've chosen? How easy is it to switch to another one?
- With which hospital or hospitals are the doctors on your insurance plan associated? If you live in a rural area, you may have only one local hospital; if you live in an urban or suburban area, there may be several hospitals from which to choose. However, the ideal situation would be that the doctor you choose is affiliated with the best possible hospital in your area—in your case, one that has a pediatric pain management program or clinic.

The Hospital

I've already alluded to your need to find a pediatrician (yes, we will get to that process soon) who is affiliated with a good hospital, and this is important because, if your child should need attention that is beyond what the pediatrician can do, the connection with the hospital is already in place. For example, if your child needs a pediatric gastroenterologist because he or she is experiencing recurrent abdominal pain, then (hopefully) your pediatrician will be able to refer you to an excellent specialist who is affiliated with the hospital. If your child should need to be hospitalized for any reason, then your pediatrician, along with any specialists he may also have on the case, will have ready access to see your child in the hospital because he has privileges at the facility. It can be difficult or more inconvenient for doctors to stay in contact with and visit patients in hospitals with which they are not affiliated.

When it comes to choosing a hospital, if you have a children's hospital in your area or a hospital that has a pediatric pain management program or clinic, any one of these would be your first choice. Many teaching hospitals—hospitals that are affiliated with a university medical school—have pain management programs for children or special pediatric units. Because these hospitals are involved in teaching tomorrow's doctors, they typically use some of the most sophisticated and up-to-date techniques and often are involved in research as well. These are advantages that can prove helpful to you and your child should he or she need specialized care.

The Pediatrician

Given any limitations presented by your insurance plan, you are now ready to find a pediatrician. In the vast majority of cases, the first medical professional who will see and evaluate your child is a pediatrician or family practitioner. Then, if she decides your child needs to see a specialist, you will be given a referral. Thus you want a pediatrician you can trust, someone you feel comfortable with, and who is knowledgeable.

If your insurance plan gives you a limited list of doctors from which to choose, you can begin your selection process from there. If you can select one from a larger pool of pediatricians, all the better. In either case, ask family, friends, neighbors, and coworkers who their pediatrician is and what their feelings are about the doctor. Hopefully some of the names you will be given are on the list from which you must choose a doctor. You can also check to see if there are any lectures or presentations being given at a local hospital or clinic or community center by a pediatrician that you can attend.

Look in your local newspaper archives for articles about area pediatricians or columns that may have been written by one of them.

Once you have a list of a few names, gather information on them by calling their offices.

- What health insurance do they accept? It's always good to ask this question, even if the doctor is on your plan's list. Also, a doctor whose name doesn't appear on your list may have been added recently and thus not appear on your information.
- Which hospitals are they affiliated with? If you have already selected a hospital, this is an important question to ask.
- Are they accepting new patients? If they are not, you can ask who is.
- Is it a private or group practice? Private practices are not as common as they used to be, but they have some advantages. Your child will always see the same doctor, and you can develop a good relationship with the pediatrician. A group practice often has more office hours and has more than one doctor available to see your child. Your doctor can also easily consult with another doctor if a question arises.
- Is the doctor board certified? Ideally, you want a board certified pediatrician, meaning that the doctor has passed the high training standards posed by the American Board of Medical Specialties (in this case, the American Board of Pediatrics; doctors can be certified in more than one specialty). It does not, however, guarantee that the doctor has a good bedside manner or that the doctor is skilled. If a pediatrician is "board eligible" or is an "active candidate for

the board," he or she has not yet taken and/or passed the board certification test but otherwise qualifies to be a board certified specialist.

- What are the office hours? Are there weekend or evening hours? What if there is an emergency?

Then there are questions you need to have answered for yourself during your visit to the doctor's office. Some information you can gather in the waiting room, such as that concerning the staff and the office environment. Other questions will be answered as you meet and interact with the doctor, whether it is for an interview or your first office visit. Bring this list with you to the doctor's office so you won't forget the types of things you should notice or the questions you may want to ask.

- How did the staff interact with you and your child?
- How did your child interact with the staff and the practitioner?
- Did the practitioner seem genuinely interested in you and your child?
- Did the practitioner answer your questions in a clear and patient manner?
- Is the practitioner open to the use of other therapies outside his realm of personal knowledge or experience? If yes, does he make referrals?
- Did the practitioner rush you through your visit? Did you feel pressured at any time during your visit to make decisions or to answer questions with which you were not comfortable?

The Assessment

The evaluation of any child who has chronic pain should include a long list of physical, psychological, and social factors. The doctor should gather information about:

- The history of the current problem (for example, when it started, location, how it varies, severity, and other characteristics). If you have kept a pain diary, it will be very useful at this point.
- The impact of the pain on the child's daily activities (e.g., eating, school attendance and performance, sleeping, social activities, sports and exercise)
- The impact of the pain on the rest of the family (e.g., is the child's condition prompting anxiety, fear, depression, or feelings of hopelessness among family members)
- History of pain problems your child and other family members have had
- Medications and any therapies—including alternative and complementary—your child is using for pain
- Your child's developmental history (e.g., when first sat up, walked, spoke) and social history (e.g., does your child have friends, hobbies or interests)
- Recent stressors in your child's life (e.g., move to a new home, new school, loss of a close friend or relative, divorce)

The doctor should also conduct a complete physical and neurological examination, which will vary somewhat depending on the complaint. Based on the doctor's findings and evaluation of the information collected, he or she may provide a diagnosis, recommend testing, or refer you to a specialist.

PAIN MANAGEMENT SPECIALISTS/CLINICS

If I had my way, every child who suffers chronic pain would have full access to a pediatric pain management clinic or, at the very least, a pediatric pain management specialist. There are dozens of pediatric pain management clinics or centers across the country, and we could use many more (see Appendix). The reason why I am so enthusiastic about pediatric pain management centers is that they typically take a multidisciplinary approach to the management of pain and offer children and their families a team of professionals who work with the child and family to understand, manage, and live with the painful situation, whatever it may turn out to be as treatment progresses.

When you take your child to a pediatric pain management center, you should get a package deal. That package should include, at a minimum: a doctor, who does the examinations and evaluations and both devises and oversees your child's treatment; a child psychologist, who guides the emotional portion of the treatment for both your child and you; and a physical therapist, who helps the child improve function or return to a higher level of functioning.

The Pediatrician

We've already talked about pediatricians in this chapter, but here we can mention that pediatricians who are affiliated with a pediatric pain management center specialize in pain management. While many other pediatricians may provide excellent general care, those who practice in such centers are more likely to be familiar with your child's specific condition and with ways to approach treatment.

Child Psychologist

I want to emphasize how critical the role of the psychologist is in the management of chronic pain in children. This is also the individual on the management team who, at least initially, is most often viewed with suspicion and even contempt by some parents. That's because some parents mistakenly believe that agreeing to talk to a psychologist is an admission that they have done something wrong or that they or their child is mentally ill.

Quite the contrary. Parents who agree to attend family therapy sessions and/or bring their child to individual therapy sessions are taking a significant and responsible step toward healing their child and their family. Because, as we will explore in more detail in Chapter 7, when a child experiences chronic pain, it's a family affair in that every member of the family is affected emotionally. A child psychologist can help provide healing guidelines for the entire family.

Another important role of the child psychologist is to perform educational testing when appropriate and to help develop a plan in concert with the school system for the gradual reintegration of the child back into the classroom if a child is missing a lot of school. Formal testing will inform both the parents and the school district of a child's performance level and will help with tailoring a custom educational program to either maintain school work on par with the child's peers or allow the child to catch up to the level at which he or she should be performing. This kind of program is called an individual educational plan, or IEP, and is discussed briefly in Chapter 8. A good psychologist not only is able to assist in the assessment of a child's educational level, but also may serve as the child's advocate with the school system in executing an effective and appropriate IEP.

Physical Therapist

Physical therapists address the musculoskeletal factors that contribute to or cause your child's pain, and help devise plans to improve physical function that has been impaired by pain and to recondition the muscles. If you are working through a pediatric pain management center, you will be referred to a physical therapist who specializes in working with children. If your physician refers you to a physical therapist, make sure it is one who is very familiar with working with young people who have your child's specific condition.

A physical therapist can develop an individualized treatment and exercise plan that fits your child's abilities and needs at home, school, and in other settings. Your child will be given exercises and coping skills to practice at home and will be expected to report back to the therapist regularly, perhaps once a week or every other week, so his progress can be monitored and any necessary changes to the treatment and exercise plan can be made.

Occupational Therapist

Occupational therapists evaluate the impact of a disease or medical condition on the activities of individuals at home, work, school, and leisure time, and then develop a plan to help them return to their previous level of activity, or as near as possible. If a child has CRPS in her hand, for example, an occupational therapist would help her with exercises so she can use eating utensils, write with a pen and pencil, button buttons, and use a computer keyboard, and will develop a program for desensitation of the hand (remember that CRPS causes exquisite pain to even light touches). Occupational therapists typically work closely with a patient's physical therapist when developing a treatment plan.

Child Life Therapist

Child life therapists are trained to show children and their families how to cope with the stress associated with their health-care experiences in a positive way and to help children deal with their pain condition according to their developmental level. This means they may use teaching dolls and books to assist children in understanding the condition they have, why they are in the hospital, or how a particular procedure will be done; show parents ways to introduce play therapy into their child's life as a way to reduce stress (see Chapter 4); and do activities, such as arts and crafts and games, with hospitalized patients to help them lead as normal a life as possible.

Not every pain management clinic or children's hospital employs child life therapists, but if you choose a facility that does, I recommend you see if their services may be helpful to you and your child.

Types of Pediatric Pain Management Facilities

I've already mentioned that a multidisciplinary pain center is the best choice for treatment of pediatric chronic pain. Such facilities offer a variety of services, including medical therapies and procedures (e.g., medications, nerve blocks), physical therapy, counseling, and other therapies such as acupuncture, biofeedback, massage, and hypnotherapy, some or all of which may be "farmed out" to other practitioners.

Many children's hospitals and other hospitals that have a pediatric unit have one or more anesthesiologists who have a special interest in pain management and who offer some pain management services. Sometimes a member of a hospital's neurology or physical medicine and rehabilitation departments will have special interests in pain management. These services may be limited to medical interventions and perhaps physical therapy. Although such services can provide very good care for some children, many children who have chronic pain need more complete treatment, including counseling and mind-body therapies.

Yet another type of pain management center is the one that offers only one or two therapies to the exclusion of nearly all others, and may also claim that its treatments are "the cure." Although the therapy offered may in fact offer some benefit when used along with other treatments, you should avoid using the services of such centers. Typically the treatments they offer are not covered by insurance and are also very expensive, which means you must pay out of pocket. There is also the chance that any treatment they offer may have a negative impact on other therapies your child is receiving, or they may even recommend you stop other treatments. Thus your safest bet is to avoid such centers.

Finding a Pediatric Pain Management Facility

Your physician may be able to refer you to a pediatric pain management facility. However, you may also want to investigate some on your own, so I've prepared a list of children's hospitals which have pain programs, clinics, and/or pediatric pain specialists. You can see the list in the Appendix.

PAIN DIARY

For some children who have chronic pain, I ask their parents to keep a diary that rates the pain from hour to hour or day to day. Keeping a written record of not only severity of pain but events in the child's life, both physical and emotional, can be very helpful when I am evaluating a child's pain and deciding on a course of action. Types of events that may be recorded are foods the child ate before experiencing an episode of abdominal pain; emotional events such as a fight with a sibling, failing a test in school, or losing a pet; and physical events such as falling off a bike.

A pain diary is useful because a person's recollection of pain isn't always accurate. However, a pain diary is useful only if it is as honest and accurate as possible. Thus parents should be diligent about filling in their child's pain diary. However, I find that compliance with diaries is poor. Many people fill them in the day before their visit to see me and they try to reconstruct all the events of the past week or two. Unfortunately, this approach often results in inaccurate and missing information, so I emphasize to parents the importance of their taking this active role in helping their child.

If the child is old enough, I may recommend that the child keep a diary, to fill it in at bedtime, and for the parents to follow up with their son or daughter to make sure the diary is completed each night. It can also be important psychologically for children to keep their own diary, as it gives them a sense of some control over their pain. In some cases, I ask both the parents and the child to keep a separate diary and for them to follow up with each other to make sure they are completed. A sample pain diary is shown in the Appendix, on page 299.

Helpful Tips for Creating a Pain Diary

- Choose a reporting form that is convenient for you. If you and your child like to use a computer, you may want to create your diary electronically and then print out the results before your doctor visit. This is a good choice for people who don't like to take notes or who have illegible handwriting. Some parents find it easier to carry around a notepad and make notes throughout the day. If your child is old enough, he or she can do the same. Yet other families keep a large calendar (with ample room to make notes for each day) on the wall in a prominent location (e.g., the kitchen or front hallway).

- Make sure you make notes at least once a day. If you put off writing down or keying in your information for days, you'll likely forget key information.
- Develop a code, if applicable. For example, if you are keeping track of certain foods that seem to be triggering migraine, you might use "P" for peanuts and "C" for chocolate.

It is also helpful to track your child's activities. In today's hectic world, many people don't realize they are filling up every moment of their lives with activities and leaving little or no down time for relaxation and stress reduction. If after school your child has Little League practice on Mondays, Wednesdays, and Fridays and games on Saturdays; has clarinet lessons on Tuesdays; and gets tutored in math on Thursdays, this is a calendar full of stressors. We will learn more about the impact of stress on pain in Chapter 7.

SUPPORT GROUPS

The healing and morale-building power of support groups cannot be emphasized enough. When children who live with chronic pain and their parents want to find others who speak their language, who truly understand what it means to stay up all night with a child who is crying with pain, or to be a teenage girl who can't keep up with her friends because of chronic pain and fatigue, or to watch your child struggle with chronic daily headaches or debilitating leg pain, they can turn to one or more of the hundreds of support groups around the country, and even around the world. Now that so many people have access to the Internet, many individuals don't have to leave their homes to find an empathetic ear or someone with whom to share their feelings and thoughts about their chronic pain or that of their child.

One of the most important things a support group can do for a child is to help him or her feel accepted and less alone. While children are growing physically, they are also developing mentally and socially, forming a sense of self. Children who feel different from their peers, who say they feel "weird" or "like a freak" because they have a condition that may keep them from being able to participate in activities with other children their age, need reassurance that they are okay, that there are other children who share their challenges. Support groups can offer these critically important character and psychological boosters.

Types of Support Groups

Basically there are two types of support group structures: self-guided and professionally guided. Self-guided support groups are run by group members. There may be a group leader who helps facilitate discussions, but none of the individuals in the group is a health-care professional who uses his or her expertise to control the group. Professionally guided groups are usually facilitated by a nurse, psychologist, social worker, or counselor.

Support groups also differ in their design. Some focus on one specific disease or condition, such as fibromyalgia or sickle cell anemia, while others have a broader scope, such as chronic pain or all neuromuscular diseases. The activities of support groups also differ. Some encourage people to share their personal experiences while others are designed to be more informative and may routinely invite speakers or hold workshops. Many are a combination of these two approaches.

Internet Support Groups

While many support groups traditionally still meet in church halls, neighborhood centers, and people's homes, the Internet has opened up a new way to share and get support from others. Internet support groups come in three forms:

- Chat rooms, in which you sit at your keyboard and communicate ("chat") with others in a virtual room. One benefit of chat rooms is that you get instant feedback, because chat rooms operate on "real time," meaning that the individuals you are communicating with are reading the messages you send immediately, unlike sending an email to someone and then waiting for a response. Chat rooms are the most personal form of Internet support groups.
- Electronic mailing lists, which you join and, as a member, receive and share emails with other people on the list. Such lists are like bulletin boards in that whenever someone on the list sends an email, every member sees it. Thus you can pose a question to the entire list, and then wait to see who and how many other members answer you. These lists are less personal than chat rooms.
- Newsgroups, in which lists of messages on similar topics are posted on the web page. You can choose to read any number of messages you wish or post a message of your own. This is the least personal form of Internet support group.

A word of caution about Internet support groups. Such groups offer anonymity, which can be a benefit if you or your child is shy, but you can't be sure of who is on the other end of your child's correspondence, and it is a sad fact of today's times that there are many predators in our society who prey on the naïve and vulnerable using Internet chat rooms (and children are, by definition, naïve and vulnerable). It is best to use sites that are sponsored or hosted by a well-known, respected organization and/or expert in the field. Sites for children should be monitored and facilitated by an expert, and you should familiarize yourself with and monitor any sites your child accesses. Naturally, you should respect your child's privacy, but you should make sure the site is run by a professional group or individual.

Finding and Choosing a Support Group for Your Child (and You)

The type of support group you choose will depend on several factors, such as availability of groups in your area, age of your child, access to the Internet, and what you wish to get out of the group. Basically, however, you can look for a support group in several places:

- Ask your health-care practitioner for a referral. If you have access to a psychologist or social worker, he or she will likely have some recommendations for you.
- Look in the newspaper. Many support groups list their meetings in a calendar section of the paper.
- Check your local telephone book.
- Contact a local, state, or national organization that is

dedicated to your child's disease. Such organizations often have support programs.

- Talk to other parents who have children with the same or similar conditions.
- Contact local religious organizations and community centers to see if they host support groups in their facilities.
- Search the Internet for organizations that have websites with information on support services.

We talk more about support groups in Chapter 8, where some children and parents share their experiences participating in such groups. If you want to contact some support groups in your area or on the Internet, see the Appendix for a list of contact information.

BOTTOM LINE

Finding competent, professional, empathetic help is one of the major tasks parents must undertake when they have a child living with chronic pain. This can be a relatively painless endeavor or a challenging one, depending on where you live, the resources available to you, and your insurance plan. It's my wish that every parent had access to the very best pediatric pain management facilities in the country, but even though that isn't possible, you now have information and guidelines to help you find the very best that's available for your child. The importance of finding and working with knowledgeable practitioners cannot be underestimated.

Chapter 4

USING THE POWER OF THE MIND

Different people feel pain differently. This statement may seem obvious to you, but there is a lot behind it that does not at first meet the eye. If a painful event occurs to, or if in a laboratory a painful stimulus is applied to, one hundred different people, you will get one hundred different descriptions of how much it hurts. Some of the differences in responses are related to an individual's past experience and personality. But much of the difference is related to the biochemical differences in the brains of different people.

Studies that produce images of how the brain is affected by pain have shown, for example, that individuals who are more sensitive to pain have areas of their brains that respond differently than those who are more tolerant to pain, and that there are differences in the biochemical enzymes in the nervous systems of these two groups of people. Similarly, there is a striking difference between how males and females perceive pain, a difference that is rooted not only in how little boys and little girls are raised and taught how to respond to pain, but in the very biochemistry of the brain and spinal cords of males and females, and how the hormone estrogen affects how the central nervous system processes pain information coming into it from the body.

The connection, then, between the mind (or, in anatomical terms, the brain) and the body, is not just psychological or behavioral, but is based on very real biochemistry and anatomy. As more and more research is done on the mind-body connection and as our understanding of this phenomenon grows, we also are enjoying an increasing appreciation of the power of the mind. The mind is an incredible tool, and the majority of people are able to capture that innate power and use it to their advantage, if shown how. One advantage is the management, reduction, and even elimination of pain and therefore suffering.

Once relegated to the land of "hocus pocus," at least in the United States, mind-over-matter therapies such as self-hypnosis, progressive relaxation, biofeedback, meditation, play therapy, and visualization have become mainstay approaches in many centers around the country. And some of the most exciting ways to see them work is in children.

One beauty of childhood is that kids are more trusting and accepting of new ideas. They have not yet formed deep-seated opinions, prejudices, and cynicism. This is one reason why children in chronic pain respond so well to the cognitive-behavioral therapies mentioned. In my center and in other centers across the country and around the world, we see so many children who are harnessing the power of their mind to reduce, manage, and even eliminate their pain. With the help of their physicians, child psychologists, psychiatrists, occupational therapists, and parents, these children are taking back some control of their lives and enjoying their childhood more.

In this chapter, I will explain the power of the mind and, through stories from my experience, share the startling ability of children to be distracted from pain. We will discuss how these cognitive-behavioral therapies work and how you, as parents, can incorporate some of them at home.

BIOFEEDBACK

Biofeedback is a technique to relieve pain that trains people to have some control over physical functions that are normally beyond our conscious control, such as heart rate, skin temperature, muscle tension, and brain waves, all without the use of drugs. Instead, patients use the power of their mind to take control of these bodily processes and then monitor their progress by looking at or listening to "feedback" from a biofeedback device that measures those functions and tells children how they are doing. Over a period of time, usually five or more sessions, depending on the condition and its severity, children can be taught to control certain bodily functions and get their body to respond in a way that reduces or eliminates the pain they've been feeling. Once they learn how to achieve this with a biofeedback machine to help them, they can slowly learn to do it without the machine, anywhere and any time they need pain relief.

Biofeedback at Work

Several different biofeedback techniques are available to help children who are in pain. For example, let's say your child is like Marc, a thirteen-year-old boy from central California, who suffers with chronic headache, one of the pain conditions that typically responds well to biofeedback. Marc had been experiencing chronic headaches for more than six months and had tried various medications without much relief. After seeing three different doctors, a fourth one recommended that Charlene, Marc's mother, take him to a pediatric pain clinic. That's when I first met him.

After a thorough examination and a talk with Marc and Charlene, it became apparent that Marc was a bright, articulate, but very tense young man. Charlene indicated that although one of the doctors had suggested that Marc try "relaxing more," he hadn't prescribed any specific techniques, so nothing had been done except to write more scripts for medications. I talked about some structured ways Marc could learn to relax, such as visualization, biofeedback, meditation, and self-hypnosis, and Marc showed some interest in biofeedback. He agreed to try some sessions, along with some individual psychotherapy.

There are several types of biofeedback, and the one we chose for Marc involved a machine called an electromyograph. An electromyograph picks up electrical signals from the muscles of the patient, who wears one or more sensors (tiny pads that are gently taped to the skin) on different parts of the body. The signals are then transmitted to a central processor. The processor emits beeps whenever the person's muscles are tense, but as the individual tries to relax, the beeping slows down. Eventually, the beeps will disappear when the muscles are relaxed.

When Marc went in for his sessions, he sat in a comfortable chair and waited while the sensors were attached to his shoulders and chest. A biofeedback technician worked with him at each session to find ways for Marc to relax the tension in his body and to hear his progress come back to him from the processor.

Marc discovered that guided imagery, visualization (see "Visualization/Guided Imagery" in this chapter), and deep breathing were effective for him. "It was kinda cool," Marc said.

"When the machine would keep beeping, I would breathe real deep breaths and then I'd concentrate real hard on how I'd be surfing these huge waves in Hawaii [Marc had surfed in Hawaii on vacation last year] and how great it felt. I could even imagine I could smell the ocean and hear the waves roaring around me. Then the machine wouldn't beep as much, and pretty soon it stopped."

Over a period of seven sessions done over four weeks, Marc was able to reduce the number of "beeps" from a steady stream to intermittent, and then to zero. Part of Marc's treatment also included talking with a psychologist about ways to use his newly learned skill in his everyday life to reduce his stress level and how to identify those elements in his life that were stressful.

Marc "graduated" from his biofeedback sessions and was then able to use his skills anywhere, anytime he felt stressed. Charlene reports that Marc still has some headache pain, but is able to manage it rather well using biofeedback and "only occasionally" needs medication.

Treating Other Conditions with Biofeedback

The biofeedback technique Marc used is effective for tension headache, migraine, fibromyalgia, recurrent abdominal pain, endometriosis, sickle cell anemia, and cystic fibrosis. Another type of biofeedback involves using a temperature monitor. This approach, which is often used for headache, migraine, and complex regional pain syndrome, is based on the fact that people's hands tend to become cold when they are under stress or in pain. If people can train themselves to change their blood flow so their hands become warm, they can relieve tension and pain at the same time. As in Marc's case, children are asked to try different ways to relax, such as visualization or deep breathing.

Juanita, a sixteen-year-old junior in high school, turned to biofeedback to treat CRPS in her right arm. Her pain had started about three months after she fell off the parallel bars in gym. Because she was right handed, the pain was making it difficult, and sometimes impossible, for her to do her school work, and she had given up her place on the gymnastics team at school as well. The arm was often so blue and cold that she was embarrassed and would wear long sleeves, even when it was hot outside.

When Juanita went to her first biofeedback session, her arm was so cold the monitor didn't even register the temperature. By the end of the second session, she was able to raise the temperature of her arm a few degrees so she could see her progress. At her fifth session, she was able to bring the temperature of her arm up to near normal, and her arm was warm and pink, and she was without pain. Juanita was able to use her biofeedback skills at school and at home without the monitor, and after more than two years of practicing biofeedback whenever she needed it, her CRPS has disappeared. There is always the possibility she will have a recurrence of CRPS, but Juanita is confident she can quickly stop the pain using her biofeedback skills.

What You Can Do

Children need to learn biofeedback skills from a professional, but once those skills are learned—in as few as four or five sessions—they should be able to use them at any time, any place they are needed. You can encourage your child to use what he or she has learned and perhaps offer to help with deep breathing, guided imagery, or visualization, and always try to provide a quiet, safe place for practice at home. (See "Visualization/Guided Imagery" in this chapter and the Appendix for guided imagery and visualization cassette tapes.)

MEDITATION

When some parents think about meditation for pain relief, they think, "my child would never sit still long enough to meditate," and for many children, this is probably true. But meditation is a proven tool in relieving chronic pain, and for some young people, especially adolescents, it is an effective one.

Defining Meditation

Some of the hesitation and skepticism that parents and children have about using meditation has to do with the fact that they don't fully understand it. Meditation is simply a way to focus the mind into a relaxed and heightened state of consciousness and perception. There are literally hundreds of ways to reach that goal, including transcendental meditation, Buddhist meditation, and Siddha meditation, but they all share the basic concepts of stilling the mind, focusing on the here and now, and taking a "time out" from the outside world.

Although there are many forms of meditation, they all

generally fall into two basic categories: concentrative and mindfulness. In *concentrative meditation,* individuals focus on something repetitive, such as breathing, a sound (e.g., a mantra), or an object (e.g., a candle flame). When people concentrate solely and completely on what they have chosen, not only does the mind become still, but physical changes can take place as well. Scientific research into concentrative meditation shows that it can reduce heart rate, breathing rate, and oxygen consumption.

Mindfulness meditation can be likened to watching a passing parade, in which the parade participants are your feelings, thoughts, and sensations, and which you let march by without thinking or worrying about them, or judging them in any way. In mindfulness meditation, you are a passive observer of your own life.

Meditation in Action

It takes a highly motivated individual to do meditation. Such an individual is sixteen-year-old Michael, who suffers with migraines. Michael became interested in meditation after he saw a video about how some children were able to deal with severe cancer pain when they meditated. "I figured if they could do it, so could I," he said. Michael and his psychologist discussed different meditation techniques, and Michael found that focusing on his breathing worked best for him. He explains:

"I get one or two migraines a month, and I know when they're coming on, because I yawn a lot an hour or two before the pain starts. If I'm home, I go into the basement, where I set up a corner with pillows. It's real quiet down there, and I can meditate without anyone bothering me. If I'm at school, I use a little room off the teachers' lounge. Then I meditate for about a half hour, and even though it doesn't completely stop the pain, at least it's not as bad, and it doesn't last as long as it used to before I started to meditate."

Michael's method is simple: he sits comfortably in a darkened room where no one will disturb him. He begins by practicing deep breathing (see box): taking several slow, deep breaths, inhaling through his nose, holding the breath for a few seconds, and then exhaling through his mouth to a count of seven. After he has taken a few deep breaths, he returns to normal breathing and focuses completely on nothing else.

"I concentrate on the sound of the breath as it goes into my nose, and then on how my chest moves as I inhale, and then on the sound as the air goes out of my nose. After a few minutes, I feel like I'm in a trance. I feel so relaxed, and the pain starts to fade. It's pretty unreal, but it works."

Michael practices meditation at least once a day, but several times a day when he's especially tense or he feels a migraine coming on.

How Meditation Works

As numerous studies have shown, meditation relieves muscle tension, which contributes to pain. It helps people achieve feelings of calm and peace and gives them a feeling of overall well-being. Meditation can also relieve the anxiety that comes with chronic pain and changes a person's emotional response to their pain. "I used to get anxious when I began to yawn, because I

DEEP BREATHING EXERCISE

This exercise can be used alone to relax anytime during the day, or as an introduction to self-hypnosis, visualization/ guided imagery, biofeedback, progressive relaxation, or meditation.

1. Place the tip of your tongue against the ridge behind and above your upper front teeth. You should keep your tongue there throughout the entire exercise.
2. Exhale through your mouth, completely releasing any air in your lungs.
3. Inhale deeply and slowly through your nose to a count of five. Keep your mouth closed.
4. Hold your breath for a count of seven.
5. Exhale through your mouth to a count of seven.
6. Repeat steps 3, 4, and 5 for a total of four to six breaths.

knew the migraine was coming," says Michael. "Even though I was taking verapamil [a beta-blocker; see Chapter 6] to prevent the pain, it wasn't enough. But now I feel I can count on meditation to get me through the pain. It makes me feel like I have some control over the pain."

Some experts believe that meditation can cause actual physical changes in the body that then control the physical sensation of pain. The theory is that meditation acts like a natural painkiller and stimulates the inhibitory nerves that extend from the brain to the spinal cord, where they stop the sensation of pain.

Treating Other Conditions with Meditation

Meditation can be helpful in children who have back pain, cancer pain, chronic tension headache, complex regional pain syndrome, facial pain, fibromyalgia, juvenile rheumatoid arthritis, and sickle cell anemia.

PLAY THERAPY

It's been said that a child's play is as serious to him or her as an adult's work is to an adult. In that case, play therapy is real serious business that's sandwiched in fun. Play therapy is the use of activities such as art projects, acting, music, dancing, or games, to desensitize or educate children about their pain. When it is used to desensitize children who live with chronic pain, play therapy acts as a distraction. This is something you can do at home to help your child deal with chronic pain.

When therapists use play therapy to educate children, it can help them better understand why they have pain or provide them with more effective ways to deal with it. Play therapy is also used to show children how a painful procedure works, such as a lumbar puncture (spinal tap) to take fluid from the spinal column, or the insertion of an intravenous line.

Child Life Therapists

The ability to engage in play and to lose oneself in playful activities is something children generally do very well. We adults, however, tend to shed our "childlike" ways or, at the very least, tuck them away and bring them out only on rare occasions. That's why when we want to engage children in play therapy as a way to reduce their pain or help them understand it better, we sometimes bring in child life therapists (see Chapter 3). Child life therapists can not only use play therapy to help your child, they can also show you as parents how to engage your child in play therapy at home and thus make you part of the treatment process.

Bradley's Story

Bradley is a bright, quiet six-year-old who had a glial tumor, the most common brain tumor in children. The tumor had been causing Bradley to suffer with severe headaches, nausea, and vomiting. His parents, Thom and Catherine, met with a child life therapist immediately after they got the diagnosis, because they were told that Bradley would need to undergo surgery, likely followed by chemotherapy, and they wanted some guidance on how to talk to Bradley about his disease and the hospitalizations he would need.

Janice, the child life therapist, sat down with Bradley and his parents and asked Bradley if he wanted to learn about what the doctors wanted to do to help him get better. Bradley didn't look too sure, so Janice asked him, "Are the doctors going to help fix the boo-boo you have inside?" When Bradley answered, "I guess," Janice removed a four-foot-long boy doll from her "Magic Box" and said, "This is Timmy, and he has a boo-boo just like yours. Would you like to help fix Timmy?"

For about thirty minutes, Janice and Bradley "worked" on Timmy. Janice showed Bradley how to give Timmy "dream medicine" through a tiny mask, and explained that dream medicine lets you sleep so you don't feel any pain. Janice then showed Bradley how to tape a tiny straw to Timmy's arm where he would get water to help his body. Next, she drew a small square on Timmy's head and said, "this is the door the doctors will use to take away the boo-boo." As Janice explained each procedure, she asked Bradley several times, "is this going to hurt Timmy?" and Bradley said no. "And why won't it hurt Timmy?" asked Janice. "Because he took dream medicine."

Janice then told Bradley that when he was ready to stop dreaming, she and his parents would be there to talk with him and make him feel better. She explained that they could draw pictures, play games, and do other fun activities.

It was important for Thom and Catherine to sit in on this and subsequent sessions Janice had with Bradley so they could learn how to talk about Bradley's condition with him. One hint Janice gave to Bradley's parents was to watch their choice of words. "I could have said to Bradley, 'the doctor will give you medicine to put you to sleep,' but if he associated being put to sleep with a family pet that had been put to sleep, then Bradley would have thought he was going to die. Naturally, an older child would have understood the phrase, so I help parents use age-appropriate language when they talk to their child and also coach them on how much information to give and how to play with their child to distract them from pain."

How to Use Play As Distraction

Using play as a distraction from chronic pain or a painful procedure can allow the child to take control over the pain and may even reduce the need for medication. Although distraction doesn't work for all children, generally young people are more easily distracted than are adults. One only has to watch children play a favorite video game to witness such intensity and disregard for their surroundings. (This type of focused concentration is actually a hypnotic state, as we discuss in "Self-Hypnosis.")

The tools you can use to distract your child from either a painful procedure or chronic pain depend on the age of your child, what fascinates or captures your child's attention, the duration of the pain, and where the distraction is taking place. If a three-year-old needs to have a blood sample taken in a doctor's office, this is a short procedure, so the distraction can be simple but must allow him or her to remain still and seated. You may, for example, try blowing bubbles or singing a favorite song with the child. An eleven-year-old child who is dealing with a flare-up of CRPS, however, needs more sophisticated and longer-term distractions, such as playing a video game or assembling a model.

What thoroughly distracts one child may have little or no effect on another. You know your child best: what captures his or her attention? Naturally, you'll need to consider the child's age and any physical limitations. Some children can even devise their own distraction plan (see box, "Liz's Plan"). Here are some suggestions you and your child can consider when you need to distract your child from pain.

- Playing an instrument, such as a guitar, drums, or kazoo. Children who choose a wind instrument can imagine they are "blowing out the pain" (though I hope for your peace and quiet they don't choose the trumpet).

- Drawing or painting. Children can depict their pain in artistic form.
- Singing along with favorite songs. Try a karaoke machine.
- Dancing, be it free-form, jazz, ballet, or hip-hop
- Watching music videos
- Writing a short play and then acting it out. Your child can give you a part too!
- Playing computer games
- Doing jigsaw puzzles
- Writing songs, both music and words
- Making figures out of clay
- Stringing beads and making jewelry
- Making cookies or cupcakes and decorating them
- Learning yoga (children's yoga studios have become popular in some parts of the country)

How Much Information Is Too Much?

Part of the job of a child life therapist is to determine a child's maturity and anxiety levels and then decide how much information should be shared with the child. In Bradley's case, he had been to the hospital several times for tests and he was familiar with his doctors. He also was a very bright child, and Janice noted that he helped her with Timmy with a quiet intensity, which led her to believe that explaining the removal of the "boo-boo" was appropriate for Bradley to hear.

Children should also be assured that it's all right to feel afraid, and that often you, their parents, are afraid too. Some parents become so distressed and anxious about what to say to their child about the pain, surgery, or a medical procedure that

LIZ'S PLAN

Liz, an extremely bright and vivacious ten-year-old child, developed her own distraction plan to help her deal with her CRPS in her foot. Here I want to share with you the plans and steps she devised for "What to do when my foot hurts." Devising this plan not only gave Liz a specific way to deal with her pain, it also made her feel she has some control over her condition.

Step 1: Keep sock on. Keep shoe on. Keep foot flat on the ground!

Step 2: Distract myself. Choose from: games, movies, candy, reading, talking about fun things with my friends, see my animals and pet and hold them.

Step 3: Relax. Practice guided imagery, deep breathing, muscle relaxation.

Step 4: Go back to what I was doing before starting step 1.

Plan A: Do 10 minutes of steps 1, 2, and 3, then do step 4.

Plan B: (In school). Go to the nurse's office for 10 minutes, then try step 4 when back in class.

Plan C: (In school). Go to the library for 10 minutes and talk to the librarian or read. Then go back to class and do step 4.

they break down. Children can take this as a sign that something dire is wrong, even when that's not true. This is where child life therapists can provide tips and guidelines on what to say to your child.

PROGRESSIVE RELAXATION

Progressive relaxation is a technique by which you gradually and systematically relax different parts of the body until the entire body is relaxed. Although there are several different ways you can do progressive relaxation, the goal is the same: release of tension from contracted muscles. It is easy for you to do at home with your child and requires no special equipment. Even children as young as three years old can understand and benefit from this exercise.

Progressive relaxation is taught by some psychologists and instructors of different disciplines, including yoga and meditation. You can get self-help tapes as well (see Appendix). We explain one popular method below, an approach thirteen-year-old Tanya uses often to help her manage her headaches.

Tanya's Story

Tanya is an energetic youngster who excels in school and belongs to the drill team, debate club, and dance club. Her headaches began about six months ago, at the beginning of the school year. At first her parents were not too concerned, as Tanya kept insisting she was all right and she wanted to go to school. She was taking acetaminophen every day, but eventually the medication didn't work. She became overwhelmed with the pain and was staying home one to two days a week. It became difficult for her to participate in all the activities she so loved, and her school work began to suffer. That's when her mother brought her to see me.

We conducted a thorough physical examination and found nothing amiss. Her chronic use of acetaminophen was behind her current chronic daily headache, although it had not been the reason her headaches had started originally. Tanya's parents welcomed a chance to speak with a child psychologist, and her assessment was that Tanya was a strong-willed child who wanted desperately to succeed but who grew very anxious and tense when she did not. Her inability to control her headaches angered her, and she had tried for months to keep going on with her activities and school work despite the pain. When the pain finally got the best of her, she felt that she had failed.

While we tapered her off acetaminophen, the psychologist suggested Tanya try progressive relaxation several times a day. This approach, she stressed to Tanya, would give her control over the amount of tension in her muscles, and once she released the tension, she could also release some of her pain.

Tanya began practicing progressive relaxation six to eight times a day. At the same time, her use of acetaminophen was replaced with use of a low-dose antiseizure medication. Her mother spoke with Tanya's teachers and principal, and she was given permission to use a private office at school for her relaxation exercises if she felt a headache coming on or was having difficulty coping with the pain. Tanya continued to see the psychologist to learn ways to better deal with stress and to not demand so much of herself, and today she experiences headache only a few times a month, which she controls with progressive relaxation.

Progressive Relaxation in Action

Below is the approach Tanya uses. Feel free to modify it to suit your child's needs. Choose a comfortable location; this exercise works best if your child is lying flat on a firm surface such as an exercise mat or lying back in a recliner. Make sure your child is wearing comfortable clothes and no shoes. You can use the following format to coach a young child, or let an older child read it through several times and let him or her do it alone. You can also tape the exercise on cassette so your child can listen to it.

- Close your eyes and place your arms by your sides. Take five slow, deep breaths through your nose, holding each one for about 5 seconds before you let it out slowly through your mouth.
- Concentrate on your feet. Tighten up the muscles in your toes by curling them under. Hold the tension for 5 to 10 seconds, then relax your toes. Take a deep breath through your nose, hold it for 5 seconds, then release it slowly through your mouth. As you exhale, imagine the tension from your toes is being released.
- Tighten the muscles in your legs and hold the tension for 5 to 10 seconds, then relax your legs. Take a deep breath through your nose, hold it for 5 seconds, then release it slowly through our mouth. As you exhale, imagine the tension from your legs being released.
- Tighten the muscles in your abdomen; hold, relax, breathe, and release as you did above.
- Tighten the muscles in your buttocks; hold, relax, breathe, and release.
- Tighten the muscles in your hands by making a fist; hold, relax, breathe, and release.
- Tighten the muscles in your arms; hold, relax, breathe, and release.

- Lift your shoulders up tight toward your ears; hold, relax, breathe, and release.
- Tighten your facial muscles—pretend you just ate a lemon; hold, relax, breathe, and release.
- Roll your neck gently from side to side and to the front; breathe and release.
- Take five deep breaths through your nose and release each one slowly through your mouth.

This entire process takes only about 5 minutes and can be done as often as needed throughout the day.

Other Uses for Progressive Relaxation

Progressive relaxation can be helpful for any child who has chronic pain to help relieve the tension and stress that typically accompany it. However, in addition to headache, progressive relaxation can be especially effective in children who have fibromyalgia, recurrent abdominal pain, cancer, sickle cell anemia, juvenile rheumatoid arthritis, and CRPS.

SELF-HYPNOSIS

Hypnosis is an altered state of consciousness or of intense focused attention during which the mind is more open to suggestion than usual. While people are in a state of hypnosis or self-hypnosis, they can learn to change their attitudes, feelings, and thoughts about pain and thus better control it.

Have you ever watched children play video games and notice that they are so mesmerized by the game they are not aware of anything else around them? They are in a hypnotic state. As adults, we may find that level of concentration harder to achieve, but most children are especially good at it. In fact, in the 1970s researchers observed that children were easier to hypnotize than adults and that self-hypnosis could be used to help them with both physical and behavioral problems. Thus self-hypnosis can be particularly useful for children when it comes to controlling pain.

Ashley's Story

Since age eleven, Ashley, now twelve years old, has been living with CRPS. The initial injury had been very minor, as is usually the case: she had tripped and hit her lower leg on the edge of a table, and she had experienced pain that was out of proportion to the injury. The pain was so debilitating she had difficulty walking. She was finally admitted to the hospital and underwent surgery for what doctors thought was compartment syndrome (a condition in which there is increased pressure within a muscle compartment—group of muscles surrounded by fascia—which causes a decrease in blood supply to the affected muscles). The surgery was successful, Ashley recovered, and she was soon able to return to her normal activities.

Several months later, however, she and a group of boys and girls were playing and she got hit in the leg with a basketball one of the boys threw at her. Once again she began to experience severe pain, even though the doctors could not find any reason for it. Despite taking opioids and undergoing an epidural nerve block (see Chapter 6), she still reported severe pain and stopped going to school.

It was at this point that Ashley's mother, Bridgett, a single mom, brought her daughter into our facility after she was referred by another physician. Because Ashley's pain was severe enough to keep her out of school, I recommended she be hospitalized. There we placed a catheter that delivered pain killers into her spine for several weeks while Ashley also participated in intensive physical therapy to help build strength and tone, and psychotherapy.

During psychotherapy it became apparent that Ashley was very attached to her mother, so much so that their roles seemed to be switched: Ashley was sometimes "mothering" her mother. Bridgett used Ashley as her confidante for her personal life and treated her as a friend rather than a daughter. Ashley had few real friends her own age, and Bridgett seemed to be taking the place of those missing friends. While most twelve-year-old girls are pulling away from their mothers and beginning to assert their independence, Ashley was drawing even closer. This unusual bond between daughter and mother is common among girls who have CRPS, and so working with a psychologist to redefine the role of child and mother is a critical part of the treatment process.

Almost immediately after we placed the catheter, Ashley's leg became pink and warm, and she was able to move without pain. After three weeks, the catheter was removed and she was sent home. We were confident that Ashley would be pain free for months, if not years, as many children are who have received medication through a catheter. Unfortunately, Ashley's pain returned within a few weeks, and Bridgett took her to another hospital, where Ashley was given oral and then intravenous opioids. Bridgett also decided to discontinue the psychotherapy sessions.

When the opioids failed to bring sufficient relief, Bridgett again brought Ashley to our hospital, where our goal was to get her off the opioids and back in school, which she had not been attending for several months. During this hospitalization, we again tried a catheter, but this time without success. We did see hope, however, as it became very obvious that Ashley's painful episodes were related to her emotional state. On the days her mother didn't come to visit her (Ashley and her mother live several hours' drive from the hospital), Ashley's leg would be pain free and look normal. Often when her mother came, however, Ashley's leg would turn blue and cold, and she was very stressed. Other situations would also cause Ashley stress, such as when she had trouble with her schoolwork (she was continuing her studies at the hospital), and her leg would flare up again, or if she became overwhelmed by feelings of hopelessness.

Gradually, the psychologist and I helped Ashley see the link between her stress level and the pain. I explained the physical part of the link: how CRPS affects the autonomic nervous system and causes some parts of the body to overreact to certain triggers, such as stress. I asked her how she felt when she was anxious, and she said her heart beat fast and her palms got sweaty. I then told her that with people who have CRPS, stress can also cause another reaction, like when her leg gets blue, cold, and painful. The good news, I said, is that she could learn how to control her reaction to stressful situations, and that would in turn control her pain. Would she like to try some stress management tools?

Ashley reluctantly agreed, and she was introduced to self-hypnosis. She had amazing success after just one self-hypnosis session. Although she had limped into the session, she walked out pain free and feeling very impressed, indeed empowered that she herself could affect her disease. The psychiatrist supplied Ashley with several self-hypnosis cassettes to use at home, and she was still pain free two months after that first session. She and her mother continue their work with the psychologist to work on their relationship issues and their link to Ashley's pain.

How Does Self-Hypnosis Work?

Children can learn to self-hypnotize after working with a hypnotherapist for one or two sessions. Preparation for self-hypnosis begins with the professional helping the child learn how to use relaxation techniques (e.g., deep breathing, progressive relaxation) and visualization to enter into an altered state of consciousness. (There are cassette tapes you can get that will help your child at home to reach this state.) Once the child is in an altered state, the hypnotherapist makes suggestions that focus on changing the severity or level of pain or on eliminating the cause of the pain.

For example, sixteen-year-old Hailey suffers with endometriosis that keeps her home from school at least two days every month, and barely functioning for several more days. She was getting minimal relief from medication, and she had a dire dread of needles, so acupuncture was not an option she would consider. After she heard that another teen with endometriosis had had success with self-hypnosis, Hailey said she was willing to give it a try.

Hailey's hypnotherapist worked with the suggestion that whenever Hailey felt the beginnings of pain in her pelvic area, she would imagine herself swimming effortlessly through a clear pool of water (Hailey had been part of her high school swim team until endometriosis sidelined her), her body weightless and pain free. As she swims, she is shedding her pain behind her, allowing it to leave her body through her feet as she cuts gracefully through the water.

Is Hypnosis Safe?

Despite the fact that hypnotherapy is widely used and recognized as a legitimate therapy for many different medical conditions, some people still believe popular myths about hypnosis. Let me assure you that hypnotherapy is a safe and effective treatment approach and that it does *not:*

- make the individual forget what has happened while in a hypnotic state
- allow the hypnotherapist to control the individual's mind
- make people do things that are against their will or beliefs
- make people fall asleep

In fact, hypnotherapists have been very successful in working with children and teaching them self-hypnosis so they can control pain and other symptoms, as we saw with Hailey.

Other Uses for Self-Hypnosis

Studies show that self-hypnosis can also be useful in reducing the painful cough, shortness of breath, and other symptoms experienced by children who have cystic fibrosis. Children with migraine have successfully controlled their pain using self-hypnosis, and many studies show its effectiveness in helping children with cancer pain, especially for dealing with the side effects of chemotherapy and painful procedures, such as lumbar puncture and bone marrow aspiration. Children with sickle cell anemia also can find relief when using self-hypnosis.

Finding a Hypnotherapist

If you are not already working with a pain management center that has a hypnotherapist, you can find one on your own. There are hypnotherapists who specialize in working with children; these pediatric hypnotherapists typically can teach a child self-hypnosis after only one or two sessions. When shopping for a pediatric hypnotherapist, you should look for one who is experienced in working with the type of pain condition that affects your child.

Hypnotherapists may be physicians, psychologists, formally trained practitioners, or informally trained individuals. To locate a certified hypnotherapist, you can begin your search with the American Society of Clinical Hypnosis (ASCH; www.asch.net), which has strict certification criteria for professionals who practice hypnotherapy (see Appendix).

VISUALIZATION/GUIDED IMAGERY

How often have you heard someone say, "that kid has a real active imagination," or "you wouldn't believe the imagination my kid has"? A vivid imagination can be a useful and effective tool when it comes to easing pain in children. When children are guided or coached to visualize specific events and circumstances, studies show that they can bring their pain under control.

Visualization and guided imagery are two sides of the same coin. Some children like to think of visualization as being the gas and guided imagery as the vehicle. Visualization is the use of positive images—as well as smell, touch, sound, and taste—during meditation or an altered state of consciousness to bring about a desired result, such as pain relief and relief from tension.

Guided imagery involves taking the objects, scenes, and other images you conjure up during visualization and using them to heal your body. For example, you may visualize sitting on a sandy beach in the Bahamas, and that may be a positive image for you. However, you can then "guide" your image and turn it into an entire story designed to relieve pain, as you can see in "Monica's Story" below.

Children are better than adults at using visualization and guided imagery because they are more comfortable using their imagination. Visualization and guided imagery are fun; they're therapy without poking and prodding or swallowing pills.

Visualization and Guided Imagery Exercises

Children can be shown some simple visualization and guided imagery exercises that they can use on their own whenever they need to manage pain and relax. It's helpful to tape several visualization or guided imagery exercises on cassette, or you can purchase commercial tapes.

Following are a short visualization and a guided imagery exercise you can use and tape. The visualization is especially easy to remember, and your child may want to use it at home, at school, or whenever the need arises.

If you decide to tape the guided imagery exercise for your child, follow the instructions that are in parentheses as you make the tape. Use a calm, soft, yet firm voice without too much inflection. You may choose to prepare the tape with low music playing in the background; nature sounds like rustling leaves and running water also work well.

Color Visualization

- Get into a comfortable position in a place where you will not be disturbed.
- Close your eyes.
- Think of a color that makes you feel relaxed and happy. Pretend that color is in the air all around you.
- Take a deep breath, breathing in slowly through your nose.
- See the color you have breathed in going into your nose, down your throat, into your chest, into your stomach, down your arms and into your fingers, down your legs and into your toes. You are full of the color. You are totally relaxed.
- Slowly release the color through your mouth as you exhale. See the color swirl out into the air around you, blending with the rest of the color.
- Now, breathe normally, and with every breath you take in, see yourself being filled with the color you have chosen. See how it fills you with peace and calm.

- Now, with every breath you let go, see the color rejoining the color that surrounds you, keeping you calm and peaceful from the outside.
- Repeat breathing in, breathing out, for several minutes.
- When you are ready to stop, take a deep breath through your nose, hold it for 5 seconds, then release it slowly through your mouth.
- Open your eyes.

Guided Imagery Exercise

- Make yourself as comfortable as possible in a place where no one will disturb you.
- Take a deep breath through your nose, hold it for several seconds, and then release it slowly through your mouth.
- I am going to count backwards from ten, and with each number you will become more and more relaxed.
- Ten, you are breathing softly through your nose and gently releasing it through your mouth (pause for 3 seconds).
- Nine (pause for 3 seconds), you may close your eyes; eight (pause for 3 seconds), seven (pause for 3 seconds).
- In your mind, imagine you are in a place that is very special to you. It may be a beach, a tree house, Disneyland, in a castle (pause 3 seconds).
- Six (pause 3 seconds), five (pause 3 seconds). In your mind, imagine you are in this place with special friends, or you may be by yourself, whichever you choose (pause 3 seconds).
- Four (pause 3 seconds). Imagine what this special place smells like (pause 3 seconds); imagine what you can hear around you (pause 3 seconds).

- Three (pause 3 seconds); reach out in your mind and touch the things around you (pause 3 seconds).
- Two (pause 3 seconds); you will remember this place whenever you need to return to it (pause 3 seconds).
- One (pause 3 seconds); you are completely relaxed (pause 3 seconds); your breathing is slow and easy.
- See yourself completely in your special place (pause 3 seconds). Look around you, smell, touch, taste, and hear everything around you. This is your special place. (Pause for 3 minutes.)
- When you are ready to return from your special place, you will be aware of my voice (pause 10 seconds).
- When you are aware of my voice, take a slow deep breath through your nose, hold it for 5 seconds, then release it slowly through your mouth.
- Open your eyes when you are ready.

Monica's Story

There are few things in life that eleven-year-old Monica enjoys as much as horseback riding. Ever since she's had fibromyalgia, however, she hasn't been able to ride Blossom. That is, except whenever she resorts to guided imagery to help her get through her painful days. She and her mother even made a tape of the guided imagery session she uses several times a week.

"I know the tape by heart," says Monica, "but I play it anyway because it's relaxing to hear my mom's voice. I start by closing my eyes and doing some deep breathing, and then I picture myself in the barn with Blossom. I can smell the hay and feel the reins in my hands. Then I get up on the saddle and we go out into the field. I can feel the sun on my head and back, and as Blossom walks real slow toward the woods, I imagine the pain in my body is falling off of me. All my pain is just falling to the ground and we leave it behind. And then Blossom starts to trot, and I feel the wind in my face and Blossom's mane is tickling my hands. And then Blossom starts to gallop, and all my pain is flying off of me as we go faster and faster until we actually lift off the ground. We keep galloping in the sky and I feel light and free. Then Blossom begins to slow down, and we come back to the earth and rest beside a beautiful stream. And I get off of Blossom and let her drink in the stream, and I lie down next to the stream. Then I take some deep breaths and slowly come back to my room."

Why Visualization/Guided Imagery Work

Some researchers believe they have captured hard evidence of why these mind-body approaches work. Using a special scanning technique called positron emission tomography (PET) on the brain, they have found that activity in the cerebral cortex is the same in people whether they actually experience something or whether they just have a vivid image of the situation in their mind. That means the brain sends the same signals to the body regardless of whether you are actually scraping your fingernails down a blackboard or if you are only imagining it in your mind. In either case, you may feel a tingle go up your spine, shake your head, and scrunch your shoulders in response to the "sound."

Other Uses for Visualization/Guided Imagery

Studies show that visualization/guided imagery is helpful for children who experience pain related to cancer, as well as recurrent abdominal pain, fibromyalgia, headache, migraine, sickle cell anemia, and cystic fibrosis.

BOTTOM LINE

Nearly every child we see at our facility is taught at least one of these mindful coping skills, and most of them find these approaches to be an integral part of their pain management program. Mind management techniques have many advantages, not least of which is that they give a child a sense of personal control over his or her pain. Children don't have to depend on a pill or a shot, they can be practiced just about anywhere, and (except for biofeedback in the initial stages) they don't require any special equipment.

I believe it is essential for children who have chronic pain to learn at least one of these mindful coping skills. Once they are mastered, these skills can be called upon throughout an individual's life, and for some children, pain management may be a lifelong task.

Chapter 5

TAPPING INTO THE BODY'S HEALING POWERS

While we know that the mind has incredible healing powers, the other half of the mind-body connection—the body—has some remarkable abilities as well. In fact, children's bodies are even better healers than those of adults, and this is an asset that we as medical professionals and you as parents can exploit in a positive way. In this chapter, we show and tell you how you can help your child harness the body's ability to heal and in the process, relieve and even eliminate pain.

Given the intimate connection between the mind and body, it is usually recommended that children in chronic pain who are undergoing treatment engage in several therapies—at least one from the "mind" category and one or more from the "body" category. A wonderful thing about these two groups of therapies is that they, unlike many medications, complement each other. You can mix biofeedback with physical therapy or acupuncture, and there are no side effects to worry you. They work together to help heal the body and mind.

In this chapter we explore some body therapies that have proved successful in treating chronic pain conditions in children and which complement the mind approaches we discussed in Chapter 4. Some of these therapies you can help your child with at home; others require the services of a professional. In either case, your understanding of these approaches will make you more prepared to help your child and explain the procedures to him or her and answer questions that may arise.

ACUPUNCTURE

The ancient Chinese healing art of acupuncture, which involves the placement of very fine needles into the skin at specific points known to relieve pain and other symptoms, has gained much acceptance among mainstream doctors as an effective treatment for chronic pain. I have seen it work in children of all ages (even as young as nine months old), and for a wide range of painful conditions. Many pain management centers and clinics include acupuncture as a regular part of their services.

How Acupuncture Works

Although we don't know exactly why or how acupuncture works, there are several theories. One is that the precisely placed needles stimulate the body's own natural painkillers—endorphins; another is that the needles prompt the pituitary and hypothalamus glands to produce healing hormones. Some believe the needles change how the immune system responds to pain, while others say they may change how blood, hormones, and neurotransmitters (chemicals that allow nerve cells to communicate with each other) flow through the body. This last idea may be closest to the traditional Chinese explanation, which is that the needles affect the flow of *chi,* which is the life force that

Chinese medicine believes surges through the body through channels called meridians. According to the Chinese, pain and disease are the result of a blockage in the meridians, and when needles are placed in certain spots, healthy energy flow can be restored.

Acupuncture in Action

One of the most impressive and inspirational stories about the use of acupuncture in children that I can share is the story of Abigail, who was a mere nine months old when I first saw her. She had been hospitalized virtually since birth, because she had a mitochondrial myopathy, a muscle condition in which the cells fail to generate energy. Abigail was unable to retain any of her feedings and vomited them repetitively, so she had to be fed through intravenous (IV) tubes. Her parents were desperate and pictured their child having to stay hooked up to IV feeding tubes as her only reliable source of nourishment, a method of feeding that is known to slowly damage the liver and lead to even more medical problems. Unable to control her vomiting with medications, her doctors asked our pain clinic doctors if we had any other things to offer for her treatment.

One of my colleagues suggested starting an acupuncture program that focused on placing needles at points known to stop vomiting. Abigail was treated for several days, and in less than a week her vomiting stopped. She was able to eat normally, and her parents were able to take her home after only a few more weeks of therapy.

For the next few years, Abigail continued to come to the clinic once a week for acupuncture treatments. The treatments allowed her to tolerate formula and, as she grew older, regular food. She continued to have an IV tube for occasional nutritional feeding and to take blood samples, but she was no longer dependent on daily IV feedings for nourishment.

Abigail continued to receive acupuncture treatments up until the age of three, when she died of complications of her mitochondrial myopathy. Although she did not survive, the acupuncture allowed her to live a relatively normal life at home with her parents up until her death, for which they were very grateful.

Fear of Needles

Perhaps because we started Abigail on acupuncture at such a young age, she never seemed to mind the needles at all. At the age of two, Abigail would come to our clinic, where needles were first placed in the wrists of her doll, then were placed in her wrists and feet while she held her doll. Ultimately, her mother learned how to insert the needles in her skin, which was even less stressful for Abigail. Typically, acupuncture needles are kept in place for fifteen minutes or longer before they are removed, and Abigail rarely seemed to object to us placing them. As she got older she was fascinated by the needles and even asked questions about them.

Yet one argument against the use of acupuncture in children is that they are afraid of needles and that getting them to cooperate may be difficult, depending on their age. While some children may be averse to needles, many others seem to tolerate them well. In a study conducted in Boston at Children's Hospital, 70 percent of forty-seven children treated for chronic pain with acupuncture said their treatments (which lasted as long as three months) had relieved their symptoms, and 66 percent of the children said the therapy was pleasant. Fifteen of the children were twelve years or younger, and thirty-two were thirteen to twenty years old.

The researchers for this study noted that children who suffer with severe chronic pain may be willing to experience short-term discomfort if they believe they will get long-term pain relief. There are ways to minimize any discomfort, however, such as distraction, guided imagery, and meditation, which children can practice during their treatments. Placing needles in specific points in the ears is another way to ease anxiety in children who are bothered by seeing the needles in their body.

In another study, one with 243 children (mean age, fourteen years) who participated in the Pediatric Medical Acupuncture Service program, the children were treated for six weeks, mostly for CRPS, RAP, and migraine/headache. While the children reported significant improvement in pain, they also experienced "overall improvement of well-being," as well as increased attendance at school and better sleep, all achieved without any side effects or complications related to treatment.

In this study, the researchers found that most of the children's fear of needles was overcome once the practitioners carefully explained and demonstrated the procedure to them. This, along with acupuncture's ability to provide results after just one or two treatments, helped the children tolerate the treatments very well.

Other Uses for Acupuncture

Acupuncture has proven itself to be an effective treatment for pain in children with sickle cell anemia, juvenile rheumatoid arthritis, endometriosis, cystic fibrosis (where it may stimulate respiratory function), cancer pain, headache and migraine, complex regional pain syndrome, and back pain. Although many children experience some pain relief after just one treatment, a series of treatments, often for a month or longer, are usually required for more lasting and effective pain relief. The number of treatments and length of therapy vary by patient and should be discussed with your health-care professional.

HYDROTHERAPY

The healing powers of water have been known since ancient times. Hydrotherapy is a broad term for the therapeutic use of water, regardless of the form it comes in. And it does come in many forms: hot and cold packs, saunas, whirlpools, steam for inhalation, hot and cold showers, and swimming pools. Because hydrotherapy comes in so many forms, it can be used for a wide variety of symptoms.

How Does Hydrotherapy Work?

Hydrotherapy can be applied in different forms; thus the form dictates the effect it has on the body. The water can be hot or cold, either in the form of a hot or cold compress, hot, moist sauna, warm whirlpool, or hot or cold showers. When you expose the body to changes in temperature, a part of the brain registers the fluctuations and tries to maintain a balance between heat loss and heat gain. For example, if you jump into a swimming pool full of cold water, your body will try to prevent heat loss by constricting your blood vessels. To make more heat, you will begin to shiver. At the same time, the release of thyroid hormones and adrenaline will cause your heart rate and blood pressure to rise. If instead of cold water you stepped into a sauna, your blood vessels would dilate, the hormones would not be released, and you would feel relaxed.

If you switch back and forth between hot and cold water (or hot and cold compresses or packs), your blood vessels will dilate, then constrict, dilate, constrict, and this alternating action stimulates blood flow. This approach can be used to treat headache and migraine. For example, seventeen-year-old Elliott finds that alternating between hot and cold showers, each one lasting about three minutes, helps reduce his migraine pain. The contrast in temperatures apparently interrupts the dilation and constriction of the blood vessels and provides relief.

Hydrotherapy can also use the buoyancy property of water. Children who have joint and muscle pain from juvenile rheumatoid arthritis or fibromyalgia can do their physical therapy, water aerobics, and swimming in a pool because there is no stress on their joints. In addition, warm water helps relax the muscles and helps relieve pain.

Hydrotherapy at Work

Daniel is one lively eight-year-old who gained much benefit from hydrotherapy. He was diagnosed with juvenile rheumatoid arthritis just after his seventh birthday, after his mother, Brenda, noticed he was limping. At first she thought it was because her son played soccer on a neighborhood team and had hurt his knee. The limping continued for about a week after Daniel's soccer season was over, and then Daniel stopped riding his bike. "I knew something was really wrong then," says Brenda. "Daniel loves to ride his bike every day after school, so I knew he must be in pain if he stopped riding." Brenda took Daniel to their pediatrician, who did a preliminary examination and then referred them to a pediatric rheumatologist, who made the diagnosis of pauciarticular juvenile rheumatoid arthritis.

Daniel was placed on antiinflammatory medication and a physical therapy program that included water exercises and swimming. At first, Daniel wasn't very happy with hydrotherapy, because he wanted to play soccer with his friends. "Daniel can be a very stubborn little boy," explains Brenda. "The physical therapist and I had to explain to him that the exercises and swimming would actually help him be a better soccer player; that if he did his exercises and took his medication, he could go back and play soccer and ride his bike when the pain went away."

Daniel continues to have frequent flare-ups of pain and swelling, which are managed with antiinflammatory drugs and hot compresses. Brenda enrolled Daniel in a neighborhood swimming program, and now he has friends he can swim with when he's having therapy as well as when he's not. "The hydrotherapy, especially the swimming, is a critical part of Daniel's getting better," says Brenda. "It's been important, not only physically, but mentally, because when he's swimming with friends he doesn't feel different or sick. He's one of the crowd."

Other Uses for Hydrotherapy

In addition to the conditions already mentioned, hydrotherapy can be effective in treating pain associated with backache, endometriosis, sickle cell anemia, and fibromyalgia. If your child has back pain or endometriosis, for example, use of a heat pack or moist heating pad can be helpful. For children who have juvenile rheumatoid arthritis or fibromyalgia, exercise in a warm swimming pool is excellent therapy, as it helps keep the joints loose and builds range of motion and flexibility in a supportive and non-weight-bearing environment. The heat of a sauna or whirlpool can also provide relief for children with any of these conditions.

MASSAGE

Touch is one of the most basic yet effective treatments for pain. Massage is a way to use touch to heal and provide relief from pain. The word "massage" is actually a general term that can include dozens of different approaches, but some of those are not appropriate for people who are suffering chronic pain. That's because in some forms of massage, practitioners may use a lot of pressure when massaging an injured or damaged part of the body. Massage can address the source of pain in your child and stop the painful nerve firing by improving the range of motion of the affected joints, relieving muscle tension, and treating trigger points to break the pain cycle.

How Does Massage Work?

Although there are dozens of types of massage, they all share several principles: they help improve circulation of blood and lymphatic fluid, stimulate the skin and nerve endings, release tension in the muscles, promote release of endorphins (the body's natural pain killers), and help enhance overall body functioning.

Massage at Work

In a study conducted at the University of Miami School of Medicine, researchers found that children with mild to moderate JRA respond very well to daily massage therapy. After thirty days of receiving fifteen minutes of massage per day, the children in their study reported less pain, fewer severe pain points, fewer times they had to limit their activities because of pain, and less morning stiffness. While this alone is good news, the rest of the good news is that the massage was done by the children's parents at home, after they received simple verbal and written instructions. The parents were pleased because not only was home massage convenient and cost effective, it also made them feel they were contributing to their children's treatment.

Massage can also be helpful for children who have fibromyalgia, although the massage must be performed by a therapist who understands the nature of fibromyalgia and the exquisite tenderness of many points in the body of a fibromyalgia patient. Children with cystic fibrosis also benefit from massage therapy. In one study, parents gave their child a twenty-minute massage every night for thirty days. As a result, the children felt less anxiety and had improved mood, both of which helped their breathing and eased their pain.

Other Uses for Massage

Since massage is a good way to relieve stress and muscle tension, which are part of every chronic pain condition, massage can benefit any child who is receptive to receiving this form of therapy, including those with migraine, chronic headache, fibromyalgia, juvenile rheumatoid arthritis, and recurrent abdominal pain. In children who have cystic fibrosis, massage may even help drain mucus from the lungs as well as release tension caused by deep coughing. If your health-care practitioner has not recommended massage therapy for your child, consult with him or her before you start such a program in case there are reasons why your child should not have massage, and to get referrals for qualified therapists and/or information on how to do the massage yourself.

PHYSICAL THERAPY/EXERCISE

Physical therapy and both aerobic and strengthening exercise are cornerstones of treatment for children who have chronic pain. The type and level of therapy and/or exercise need to be determined individually for each child, usually by a physical therapist, based on his or her physical condition, type of pain, and preferences. The reason preference is important is because we want the children to enjoy these activities as much as possible. Often, regular—meaning for a set number of days per week for a predetermined length of time—therapy or exercise will be a major tool in helping them fight or ward off pain, as well as keeping them flexible and toned for many years to come. Thus it's important to work with a physical therapist (and sometimes an occupational therapist as well) to determine which activities are most beneficial, effective, and fun.

It's very rewarding to see the dramatic improvements that can occur when children follow their physical therapy programs. When a child has been hospitalized for pain management and is "captive," so to speak, he or she must participate in the physical, and often occupational therapy, that the doctor has ordered. When the child goes home from the hospital, the parents are usually armed with a home exercise program and recommended activities, and the child is expected to return routinely for follow-up visits with the physical therapist to monitor progress and to make changes to the program as needed. Children who have not been hospitalized generally meet with a physical therapist one or more times a week for therapy sessions and are also given a home exercise program.

Physical Therapy at Work

I've seen hundreds of children benefit from physical therapy when they have followed the programs developed for them. One such child was ten-year-old Ruth, who had moderate to severe complex regional pain syndrome in one of her legs. Ruth's only treatments were the low-dose tricyclic antidepressant amitriptyline, given for some pain relief and to improve sleep, and physical therapy. At first, Ruth saw her physical therapist three times a week until the therapist developed an exercise routine for her to do at home. Then she would come to see her physical therapist once a week. At first, Ruth wasn't too pleased with her physical therapist and gave her a hard time as she showed her various range-of-motion exercises, which involve moving the limbs within their normal range to help keep the joints flexible and to reduce stiffness. The therapist found that she got much more cooperation once she added water aerobics to the routine, and then Ruth actually began to look forward to those sessions. Ruth's CRPS resolved with these simple measures, and so far has been in complete remission for several years.

Physical therapy is critical for children who have CRPS in order to get the affected body part functioning again. First, however, we often need to relieve the pain so the child can tolerate and participate in therapy. Sometimes in the most affected cases this means a child needs to be hospitalized for aggressive pain management, such as an epidural block or sympathetic nerve block (see Chapter 6), followed by intensive physical therapy in the hospital for several weeks, and physical therapy at home once the child is released from the hospital. For other children, an oral analgesic medication and a regular physical therapy and exercise program at home and frequent monitoring by a physical therapist are all that's necessary.

Aerobic Exercise

Working up a sweat when you're experiencing pain can provide significant pain relief. When I have a migraine, I find that hopping on my bicycle and riding hard and fast for thirty minutes or so greatly reduces the intensity of the pain. Why is that possible? Research shows that regular aerobic exercise reduces not only the number of migraine attacks, but also their intensity and the length of the attacks. And the reason it works is that the beta-endorphins, the body's natural painkillers, increase in number in the bloodstream and in the brain. You may be familiar with the phrase "runner's high," which is in fact the euphoric feeling runners can get when their endorphin levels increase as they run hard and/or long distances. This "high" can be experienced by anyone who engages in vigorous exercise.

Other Uses for Physical Therapy and Exercise

Physical therapy is an essential part of the treatment program for juvenile rheumatoid arthritis, fibromyalgia, back pain, and any painful condition in which children need assistance with strength, tone, flexibility, and range of motion. Most other children with chronic pain or chronic illness have abstained from exercise for a while, and have become deconditioned. These children will also benefit from a graded exercise program under the watchful eye of an experienced physical therapist, to restore their physical condition and muscle strength and tone. Exercise in the form of participation in competitive sports, skateboarding or riding bikes with friends, swimming, or more disciplined forms such as brisk walking or jogging, should be a part of every child's life, within safe parameters as determined by your child's doctor.

TENS

Transcutaneous electrical nerve stimulation (TENS) is a pager-sized device that delivers a mild electrical stimulation to the body to help relieve pain. A TENS unit contains a battery pack from which there are wires and electrodes that attach to the skin and transmit mild electrical impulses, which cause a slight tingling but at the same time, relieve pain.

How TENS Works

Experts are not certain exactly how TENS works, and study results differ about its effectiveness. Some say that the electrical impulses prevent pain signals from reaching the brain in a manner similar to acupuncture.* Others say the impulses distract patients from their pain, while yet another theory is that any relief is purely a placebo effect. Researchers also disagree about where to place the electrodes, although often children and their doctors find that it is a case of trial and error until the most effective spots are found.

Although we may not know how TENS works, the truth is that it *does* work for some children. Once the electrodes are

---

*Drs. Melzak and Wall described their famous "Gate Theory" of pain in the 1970s, in which they hypothesized that one set of nerve impulses coming into the spinal cord could "close the gate" on another set of nerve impulses entering nearby in the spinal cord. In this way, electrical tingling from TENS entering the spinal cord can "close the gate" on the electrical impulses coming from a nearby painful source, such as an inflamed joint, a surgical incision, or a broken bone. While purely hypothetical when Drs. Melzak and Wall developed their Gate Theory, in the subsequent decades there has been ample scientific evidence to prove the theory correct.

attached to the skin, pain relief occurs within thirty to sixty minutes in nearly 100 percent of patients. TENS is very safe, and it causes virtually no side effects. About one third of children who use TENS experience some skin irritation, mostly from the electrode gel drying out, or they react to the tape that is used to secure the electrodes to the skin.

Other Uses for TENS

Although some health-care practitioners report success treating chronic pain in children with TENS, that has not been our universal experience. However, it is an option your doctor may suggest and one you may wish to explore. Use of TENS in very young children is not recommended, as it requires some degree of maturity to be responsible for a TENS unit. In general, though, if a child has the intelligence and sophistication to play a hand-held video game, she probably has the skill to understand and effectively use a TENS unit. Virtually all insurance companies will provide reimbursement for a trial of TENS, and for the TENS unit itself if the trial proves successful.

TENS may be effective in helping relieve the pain associated with sickle cell anemia, juvenile rheumatoid arthritis, complex regional pain syndrome, endometriosis, and fibromyalgia.

BOTTOM LINE

The body therapies covered in this chapter can be used alone or, better, along with the mind approaches discussed in the previous chapter to relieve chronic pain in children. Children often respond well to mind-body therapies, and they are preferable to, as well as complementary of, any medication interventions we may need to take. I encourage you to talk to your health-care practitioners about incorporating some of these approaches into your child's treatment program.

Chapter 6

WHEN MEDICATIONS ARE NEEDED

I'm in favor of anything that allows us to reduce the number or amount of pharmaceuticals given to children. And I am so grateful that we as physicians and you as parents have many options other than drugs with which we can treat your child's pain, as you've seen in the previous chapters.

But the truth is, even though pain medications are often not the first choice when we treat chronic pain in children, often they are needed, along with other approaches. Sometimes drugs are only required for a very short time, as when they are given to help a child get started with a physical therapy program. Occasionally they are required long term, as when we are trying to prevent recurrent migraine. However, you as parents should *not* feel guilty about your child taking these drugs. When they are used appropriately and responsibly, they can be a tool to help your child reach a more comfortable level and perhaps be better able to use other pain management methods.

We live in a society in which we want a quick fix for everything: from our cars to our cell phones to our health, we want the magic potion that will make them better when something goes wrong. This is especially true when we're talking about the health of a child. This strong desire to cure our children of every illness that comes down the pike has, unfortunately, led some of us—doctors and parents—to be a bit irresponsible.

For example, up until very recently, many doctors were quick to prescribe antibiotics to children for conditions, such as colds and flu, that would never respond to these drugs. Why? Because many people believe that antibiotics can cure just about anything, when the truth is that they are for bacterial infections, not viral infections like cold and flu. Many parents would *insist* that their doctor give them a prescription for antibiotics, even if the doctor said they wouldn't work. The result is that many of these antibiotics now *don't* work for a great number of children and adults because the infections they once were able to destroy have become resistant to the drugs.

What has this got to do with giving drugs to children who live with chronic pain? It emphasizes that we need to be judicious when prescribing drugs for our children, especially since some of these children may need to manage their pain for many years—perhaps their entire lives. It reminds us that no drug is a silver bullet and that we need always to have other treatment options in our little black bag. It emphasizes that when a drug isn't effective, it should be discontinued, rather than continued while adding another drug to the treatment program. And it awakens us to the fact that if we *don't* act responsibly, unintentional harm can come to those we most want to help.

DRUGS AND CHILDREN

If you've ever read the prescribing instructions that come with prescription drugs (and over-the-counter drugs as well), you may have seen a warning something like this: "The safety and dosage of this drug have not been established for pediatric use" or "the safety of this drug has not been established for children under 12." This means that the drug has not undergone any research *by the manufacturer* to verify that it is safe and effective when given to children. In fact, according to the American Academy of Pediatrics, only about 25 percent of drugs on the market have been approved for use in children. What does this mean, and how do you know if the drug and dose your doctor wants to give to your child are safe?

When a pharmaceutical company develops a new medication, it first must prove that the medication is safe in animals, then that it is safe and effective in healthy human volunteers, and lastly that it is safe and effective in those people with the disease or condition the drug is designed to treat. The Food and Drug Administration (FDA) then reviews all the experimental data provided by the pharmaceutical company, and if the evidence of safety and effectiveness is strong and compelling, the FDA will license or "approve" the drug. However, the drug approval will only be for those specific circumstances that the pharmaceutical company has taken the trouble to study, and the drug label will reflect that. So, for example, if the company has only demonstrated effectiveness and safety in adult men with condition X, the drug approval will only be for adult men with condition X, not women with X, and not children with X.

Unfortunately, whether a pharmaceutical company decides to measure effectiveness and prove safety in children generally depends upon their judgment of the cost of doing those studies versus the expected income from selling the drug for use in children, not whether the drug is needed or useful in children. Because the size of the market for drugs for children is small and the cost of doing drug studies is high, few pharmaceutical companies have chosen to formally study their products in children or teenagers.

But that the FDA has not approved the labeling of a drug for use in children does not mean it is not safe or effective for children. Often there are many studies done not by the manufacturer of the drug, but by independent researchers who demonstrate safety and effectiveness. Other times, anecdotal experience or informal work has been done by thousands of doctors who have given the drug to their pediatric patients. These doctors know from experience what dose is most effective and safe for use in children of various ages. (See Chapter 3, "Finding Professional Help," for more on finding the right doctor for your child.)

Off-label Use of Drugs

One interesting thing about many medications prescribed for pain is that although they were originally developed to address one specific condition or symptom, say, depression, and they receive the approval of the Food and Drug Administration for that use, doctors and researchers often then find that other ailments respond to them. This is especially true when treating chronic pain.

For example, if your child suffers with chronic tension headache, your doctor may prescribe an antiseizure drug called carbamazepine or sodium valproate. Why? Because researchers have found that carbamazapine and valproate are effective against certain kinds of pain, including headache. Even though these drugs were approved by the Food and Drug Administration for treatment of seizures, doctors are allowed to prescribe drugs for other uses. These other treatment indications are called "off-label use."

You should know that off-label use of drugs is perfectly legal and legitimate, and insurance companies will cover off-label use of drugs if they are included or approved for inclusion in one or more of the following:

- American Hospital Formulary Service—Drug Information
- American Medical Association—Drug Evaluations (no longer published)
- USP Drug Information

You may want to check with your insurance company if your doctor prescribes a drug for off-label use to see if it will be covered.

Not Little Adults

It's important to remember that children are not little adults. Children respond differently to mind-body treatments for pain than adults. The same is true for medications: children's bodies are not yet fully mature, so their organs react to drugs in a different way. They also metabolize substances at different rates, and have less body mass. Your doctor must take all of these factors into consideration when she writes a prescription for your child.

Prescribing More Than One Drug

In some cases, multiple medications may be necessary when treating pain that is not responding well to single drugs. This is when doctors may prescribe an adjuvant drug—one that is used to enhance the pain-killing effectiveness of another. Often the adjuvant drug is an off-label one—approved for uses other than relieving pain, such as antidepressants, antihypertensives, and beta-blockers. We discuss these and other adjuvant drugs in the sections below.

It is difficult to know who will benefit from one adjuvant drug or another; therefore your doctor may try brief courses of different drugs to find the most effective one for your child. This approach of trial and error can be a frustrating time for you and your child, but it's important to find the medication that will provide the best benefit.

Given that introduction, we will now look at the most common categories of drugs given to children who have chronic pain, the various medications in each group, their benefits and risks, and the conditions for which they are prescribed.

ACETAMINOPHEN

Acetaminophen is a pain killer and fever reducer that affects how the brain perceives pain. Thus it can reduce the intensity of pain even though it has no direct effect on its cause, unlike anti-inflammatory drugs, which reduce the inflammation that is often the cause of or contributor to pain. For some children, acetaminophen can be an alternative to nonsteroidal antiinflammatory drugs if they are sensitive or allergic to these latter drugs. Acetaminophen is available over the counter and by prescription; it is also sold in combination forms, along with aspirin, caffeine, barbiturates, and/or opioids (see below).

Types of Pain Treated with Acetaminophen

Acetaminophen is usually used to treat mild to moderate pain associated with different conditions. However, when it is combined with other medications, it can be given to treat more severe pain. Types of pain treated with acetaminophen include:

- Back pain
- Endometriosis
- Fibromyalgia
- Headache
- Juvenile rheumatoid arthritis and other forms of arthritis found in children
- Migraine

Types of Acetaminophen

Acetaminophen is available alone or combined with other medications, which boost its pain-killing abilities.

- **Acetaminophen alone** (e.g., Dynafed, Panadol, Tylenol) is available over the counter and by prescription. For children, acetaminophen is available as an elixir and drops; it is also available in chewable tablets and caplets.
- **Acetaminophen/aspirin/caffeine combination** is sold as Excedrin Migraine over the counter. Like all acetaminophen products, it should be used with caution (see "Side Effects").

This combination in particular, however, can cause caffeine withdrawal headaches if it is used on a daily basis. What happens is that the child wakes up with a headache, caused by the caffeine from the previous day's dose having worn off. The child then takes another dose to get rid of the headache, and a vicious cycle of pain begins.

- **Acetaminophen plus an opioid** (e.g., codeine, hydrocodone, or oxycodone) is available in many forms: for example, with codeine (Tylenol with Codeine No. 2 and 3, Phenaphen with Codeine No. 3); with hydrocodone (Anexsia, Bancap HC, Dolacet, Lortab, Vicodin); and oxycodone (Endocet, Percocet, Tylox). The acetaminophen portion of the medication helps reduce pain and fever while the opioid portion helps reduce moderate to severe pain and offers a calming effect.
- **Acetaminophen plus butalbital plus caffeine** (e.g., Fioricet) can be used for migraine headache in children. The butalbital is a barbiturate sedative, and the caffeine boosts the power of the other two drugs. This combination is associated with abdominal cramps, bloating, dizziness, drowsiness, shortness of breath, and sedation. This has not been tested for safety in children younger than twelve years.

Possible Side Effects

Acetaminophen alone rarely causes side effects when it is taken as directed. This drug is not for long-term use, however, as prolonged use can cause liver damage, itching, fever, rash, yellowing of the eyes, and low blood sugar. When combined with caffeine and aspirin or caffeine and butalbital, it can cause rebound headache if taken more than two or three days a week. The opioid-combination forms may cause drowsiness, dry mouth, constipation, dizziness, lightheadedness, nausea, vomiting, shortness of breath, and urinary retention (inability to urinate).

How to Use Acetaminophen

Even though acetaminophen is available over the counter, please consult your pediatrician before giving this medication to your child. Too often people believe that because a drug is available over the counter it does not pose any danger. Acetaminophen can cause serious side effects if it is taken for a long time or in large doses, and what constitutes a safe dose for an older child or adult is likely a dangerous dose for a young child. In general, no child should ever take more than 75 mg of acetaminophen per kilogram of body weight per day, or about 35 mg of acetaminophen per pound of body weight per day. For example, of your child weighs 50 pounds, his maximum daily dose of acetaminophen should be no more than 1,750 mg per day. It is very important to read the label on the bottle of acetaminophen and do the arithmetic to be sure your child does not exceed his or her daily maximum amount, or severe liver damage could occur.

ANTIDEPRESSANTS

Antidepressants are a category of drugs composed of several different subgroups, including selective serotonin reuptake inhibitors (SSRIs) and tricyclics. Although antidepressants are used to treat depression and other mood disorders, experts have found they are also helpful in treating different types of pain, even though the reason they help to relieve pain is not clear.

Pain Treated with Antidepressants

- Cancer (neuropathic pain—caused by nerve damage—associated with cancer)
- Chronic daily headache
- Complex regional pain syndrome
- Fibromyalgia (to help reestablish sleep patterns)
- HIV/AIDS
- Migraine

Typically, it can take up to five days for antidepressants to begin providing pain relief, as these drugs need to build up in the bloodstream. When antidepressants are used to treat pain, they are usually given in addition to other pain medications and at lower doses than used to treat depression.

Types of Antidepressants

Tricyclic antidepressants are drugs that relieve pain by affecting the part of the brain that controls the pain signals that pass between nerve cells. Tricyclics that are usually prescribed for pain include amitriptyline (Elavil), clomipramine (Anafranil), doxepin (Sinequan), desipramine (Norpramin), imipramine (Tofranil), and nortryptiline (Pamelor).

Selective serotonin reuptake inhibitors (SSRIs) may help relieve pain by restoring the level of serotonin (a hormone involved in determining mood) to normal. Drugs in this category include fluoxetine (Prozac), fluvoxamine (Luvox), paroxetine (Paxil), sertraline (Zoloft), trazodone (Desyrel), and venlafaxine (Effexor). Unfortunately, the experimental evidence that the SSRIs are effective painkillers is weak. While their side effects are milder and better tolerated, generally they are less effective than the tricyclic antidepressants.

Antidepressants at Work

Several years ago, Peter and Rebecca brought in their fifteen-year-old daughter, Melissa, to see me. Melissa had been experiencing chronic abdominal pain and cyclic vomiting for about eight months. During that time, Peter and Rebecca had taken their daughter to several different doctors, who had done complete physical examinations and performed various tests, but found nothing physically wrong.

Although our examinations also revealed nothing amiss, I began to suspect Melissa had abdominal migraine when she revealed that along with the pain and vomiting, she also sometimes experienced considerable headache pain that was accompanied by aura (see Chapter 2). When I questioned her further, I learned that the abdominal pain and vomiting episodes, which occurred every four to six weeks, seemed to be associated with her menstrual cycle.

At that point, I decided to treat her as if she had classic migraine and prescribed a tricyclic antidepressant, amitriptyline, for daily use and a triptan, sumatriptan, for when the attacks occurred. Happily, her episodes of abdominal pain and vomiting were reduced to about one per year, and she is able to control that occurrence with the sumatriptan, which keeps the vomiting and pain to a minimum if she takes it as soon as she suspects an episode is coming on. Melissa is now in college, and although she still averages one episode per year, she hopes one day soon those will disappear.

Possible Side Effects

All tricyclic antidepressants share similar side effects, including drowsiness, dry mouth, low blood pressure, impaired vision, constipation, and infrequently urinary retention. Some children experience dizziness or faintness when they rise quickly from a reclining or seated position. The side effects of clomipramine and nortriptyline tend to be less severe than those associated with amitriptyline. Because all tricyclics cause some degree of sleepiness, they are usually given at bedtime. In high doses, or in susceptible individuals, heart rhythm disturbances may be caused by tricyclic antidepressants. That is why if it is necessary to increase the dose of a tricyclic beyond what I consider to be a low dose range, I get an electrocardiogram on my patients to be sure that their heart rhythm is normal and not susceptible to disturbance by their medication. One more thing to note is that desipramine has been associated with sudden death in teenagers, presumably related to the same mechanism, and for that reason this is a drug I no longer prescribe.

Selective serotonin reuptake inhibitors tend to have less sedative effect than tricyclics and no heart-related effects. Possible side effects of SSRIs do include dizziness, tremor, headache, chills, anxiety, insomnia, nausea, vomiting, diarrhea, fatigue, sweating, dry mouth, constipation, and confusion.

Because many (but not all) SSRIs commonly cause insomnia, they are generally given in the morning rather than at bedtime.

How to Take Antidepressants

Children typically metabolize tricyclic antidepressants more rapidly than adults, so your doctor may prescribe twice-a-day dosing. If your child is having difficulty sleeping or staying asleep through the night, an evening dose of amitriptyline may be helpful. However, if you want to avoid sedation, nortriptyline may be prescribed.

ANTIHISTAMINES

Antihistamines are drugs typically used to treat symptoms of allergies, hay fever, and colds, as well as hives. Off-label, they are occasionally prescribed along with painkillers as complementary treatment for various types of chronic pain.

Condition Treated with Antihistamines

The only chronic pain condition for which I recommend the use of antihistamines is the prevention of migraine.

Types of Antihistamines

There are many antihistamines on the market, but the one usually used to help relieve chronic pain along with painkillers is cyproheptadine (Periactin). Cyproheptadine is available in tablets and liquid.

How Antihistamines Work Against Pain

Antihistamines block the action of histamines, chemicals that are released during an allergic reaction, at receptor sites. They do not affect the rate of histamine release, nor do they deactivate histamine. They also have a sedating effect and can relieve anxiety, agitation, and tension, which in return can reduce pain.

Possible Side Effects

Use of antihistamines can cause tiredness, sedation, dizziness, restlessness, excitation (especially in children), ringing in the ears, aggression, nausea, and vomiting. Cyproheptadine can also stimulate the appetite and lead to weight gain.

ANTIHYPERTENSIVES

Medications used to treat high blood pressure come in several categories, including beta-blockers, calcium channel blockers, alpha-agonists, and diuretics, but they can all be grouped together under the heading "antihypertensives." Drugs in the first three categories are sometimes prescribed along with traditional painkillers to treat specific types of chronic pain in children.

Conditions Treated with Antihypertensives

- Complex regional pain syndrome
- Chronic daily headache and prevention of migraine
- Endometriosis
- Other chronic pain

Types of Antihypertensives

- **Atenolol** (Tenormin), a beta-blocker, comes in tablets. It can be taken with or without food, but taking it with food can reduce by up to 20 percent the amount of medication the body absorbs.
- **Metaprolol** (Lopressor), a beta-blocker, comes in tablets.
- **Nadolol** (Corgard), a beta-blocker, comes in tablets. It can be taken with or without food.
- **Propranolol** (Inderal), a beta-blocker, is available in tablets, capsules, and liquid, and is most effective if taken on an empty stomach. I have found it to be effective for migraine.
- **Verapamil** (e.g., Calan, Isoptin), a calcium channel blocker, comes in tablets, capsules, and as a liquid. Although it works best when taken on an empty stomach, verapamil can be taken with food if it upsets the stomach.
- **Nifedipine** (Procardia), a calcium channel blocker, is available as a tablet and in a liquid-filled capsule. This medication can be a good choice for small children because the liquid-filled capsules can be pierced and the mint-flavored liquid can be placed on the tongue.
- **Clonidine** (Catapres), an alpha-agonist, is available as a transdermal patch, in liquid, and as a tablet. Availability as a

once-weekly patch makes it easy for children to use. It is also approved for injection into the epidural space in the spine for management of cancer pain.

Typically I use the beta-blockers only for prevention of migraine and management of chronic daily headache. Children who are very active, especially those who participate in sports like soccer, swimming, and running, should not take beta-blockers because these medications limit the maximum heart rate that can be achieved by exercise, and therefore limit endurance. Beta-blockers also should not be given to children who have asthma.

I find calcium blockers to be useful for prevention of migraine and chronic daily headache, and for CRPS. The caution with calcium blockers is to watch for a rise in blood pressure, especially first thing in the morning. Some children experience dizziness or faintness when they rise quickly from a reclining or seated position, especially when they first start taking calcium blockers.

How Antihypertensives Work Against Pain

Experts believe antihypertensives may work in several ways to relieve pain. One possibility is that they cause the release of serotonin and other neurotransmitters, which reduces the sensation of pain. These drugs, especially calcium channel blockers, may also help stabilize the size of blood vessels and thus prevent them from contracting and dilating, actions which can cause pain. How clonidine works is well understood. In the spinal cord, pain nerve fibers have special chemical receptors for norepinephrine, which acts as one of the body's own painkillers. Clonidine can interact and activate that receptor, mimicking the effect of the body's norepinephrine.

Possible Side Effects

The most common side effects associated with antihypertensive drugs are, of course, low blood pressure and therefore dizziness, fatigue, and drowsiness. Headache, constipation, and stomach upset may occur in some children. Some children who take beta-blockers experience a slower than normal heart rate and thus find it difficult to participate in vigorous exercise. If your child has asthma, diabetes, heart failure, or Raynaud's syndrome, he or she should not take these beta-blockers.

ANTISEIZURE DRUGS

Antiseizure or anticonvulsant medications are traditionally used to treat people who have epilepsy or other conditions characterized by seizures. Although no one is certain why antiseizure medications help relieve pain, experts have known for many years that people who have seizures are more likely to have migraines, and vice versa, and that people with seizures who take these medications get migraine relief. Doctors also found that antiseizure drugs helped relieve other types of pain as well.

Conditions Treated with Antiseizure Drugs

- Cancer (neuropathic pain—caused by nerve damage—associated with cancer)
- Chronic daily headache
- Complex regional pain syndrome
- Fibromyalgia
- Migraine

Types of Antiseizure Drugs

Antiseizure drugs that are helpful in relieving neuropathic (nerve) pain and head pain include the following:

- **Carbamazepine** (Tegretol), available in tablets, capsules, and oral suspension. I prefer to use carbamazepine for neuropathic pain syndromes only, and only if other medications have not been effective, because this drug can cause toxicity of the liver, pancreas, and bone marrow. Children who do take carbamazepine must have periodic blood tests to monitor toxicity and drug levels, and this can be unpleasant for them.
- **Gabapentin** (Neurontin) comes in tablets, capsules, and oral solution. It is the best tolerated of the antiseizure drugs mentioned here and causes virtually no side effects in children. It is commonly used to help prevent migraine and various causes of neuropathic pain.
- **Topiramate** (Topamax) comes in tablets. Although it can be very effect for prevention of migraine, most patients report memory and thinking problems when they use this drug or, as some children have told me, "I feel stupid" when they

take topiramate. This can be a big drawback for children and their schoolwork and is a reason why this is not my first choice for a painkiller in this class.

- **Valproic acid** (Depakote) comes in capsules, tablets, liquid, and capsules containing sprinkles. Valproate can be effective in the prevention of migraine, but it also can cause liver and bone marrow toxicity and requires blood monitoring. However, in children with migraine who are hyperactive, manic, or who have difficult-to-control behavior the calming effect of valproic acid can be a good choice.

None of these drugs provides instant relief: it typically takes at least one to three weeks before your child will notice relief from these medications. However, it is important to follow your doctor's prescribing instructions and to allow the drug to build up gradually in your child's bloodstream to work effectively.

How Antiseizure Drugs Work Against Pain

The ability of antiseizure drugs to relieve pain is likely related to the way they affect the neurotransmitter gamma aminobutyric acid (GABA). This substance helps prevent nerve cells from overfiring or spontaneously firing, an activity that can cause pain and is associated with chronic pain states.

Possible Side Effects

The different antiseizure drugs share some side effects, including drowsiness and sedation. However, each one also has the ability to cause specific reactions, as shown here:

- Carbamazepine: nausea, vomiting, unsteadiness, dizziness
- Gabapentin: common in children three to twelve years are aggressiveness, anxiety, crying, euphoria, hyperactivity, and restlessness
- Phenytoin: constipation, dizziness, impaired coordination, mental confusion, nervousness
- Valproic acid: aggression, depression, hyperactivity, indigestion, nausea, and vomiting

BOTULINUM TOXIN TYPE A (BOTOX) OR B (MYOBLOC)

This "drug" is probably best known as the injection that erases wrinkles—Botox—which is sought after by many women and men who want to look younger. Yet botulinum toxin also has another use, the ability to reduce pain. Botulinum toxin is a purified protein that belongs to a class of substances called neurotoxins. This toxin is produced by the bacterium *Clostridium botulinum,* the same one that causes botulism, or food poisoning. When the toxin is diluted to a great degree and injected under the skin in minute quantities, it can do much more than help erase wrinkles: it can reduce pain.

Conditions Treated with Botulinum Toxin

- Chronic daily headache
- Facial pain

- Fibromyalgia
- Migraine

How Does Botulinum Toxin Work?

When botulinum toxin is injected into or near muscle, the muscle becomes temporarily relaxed, typically for four to six months, depending on the site. We're not certain exactly how botulinum toxin relieves pain, but there are several theories. One is that it is taken up by the nerve fibers near where it is injected, and may prevent the release of acetylcholine, a substance nerves need to cause muscle contractions and pain. Thus botulinum toxin injected into specific muscles in the forehead area may prevent muscle contractions that can trigger migraine. Another theory is that the toxin may affect the nerve signals that are involved in pain perception, thereby dulling or eliminating the experience of pain. Whatever the reason, I have seen it work well time and time again in my patients who have chronic headache or migraine who have not responded to other therapies. I have also found it helpful in children who have fibromyalgia and facial pain.

Botulinum Toxin at Work

One of the most difficult cases to come my way was Luke, a fifteen-year-old boy from Wyoming who had chronic facial pain with no apparent cause. Luke and his parents had been to numerous doctors, and none had been able to diagnose his problem. Despite more than six months of psychotherapy and various pain medications, Luke continued to suffer persistent pain that occasionally flared into severe pain. He was understandably depressed, missed a lot of school, had dropped off the school soccer team, and was unable to participate in activities with his friends.

After our examination also did not turn up a definite cause for his pain, I decided to see if Luke and his parents would be willing to try botulinum toxin injections. After we discussed the procedure and possible side effects (mild headache, mild bruising at injection sites), Luke was anxious to give it a try. I injected the toxin into several selected sites on his face, and he reported that he barely felt the needles at all. Within twenty-four hours, Luke was relatively pain free for the first time in years.

Although Luke's pain had essentially disappeared after the first treatment, Luke and his parents understood that he would need to continue getting injections, probably every four to five months, until the pain went away completely or another effective treatment could be found. Luke and his family returned to Wyoming and were put in touch with a physician there who would continue giving him the injections as needed. I also urged them to continue psychotherapy until they felt Luke's depression was resolved.

CORTICOSTEROIDS

Corticosteroids are antiinflammatory medications similar to the natural hormone, called cortisol, produced by the adrenal glands. They are usually reserved for children who have severe pain that will not respond to other medications or who can't take NSAIDs.

Conditions Treated with Corticosteroids

- Cancer-related pain
- Chronic daily headache
- Complex regional pain syndrome
- Juvenile rheumatoid arthritis and other less common arthritic conditions that affect children (e.g., systemic lupus erythematosus, ankylosing spondylitis, Reiter's syndrome, dermatomyositis)
- Migraine
- Ulcerative colitis

Types of Corticosteroids

The types of corticosteroids used to help treat pain are in a category called glucocorticosteroids and include dexamethasone, hydrocortisone, methylprednisolone, prednisolone, and prednisone.

- **Dexamethasone** (Decadron, Dexasone) can be used to stop nausea and vomiting caused by cancer chemotherapy. It is available as a tablet, which should be taken with food, as an injection, and as a syrup.
- **Hydrocortisone** (Cortef, Hydrocortone) helps relieve inflammation and pain. It is available as a tablet and in suspension.
- **Methylprednisolone** (Medrol) is available in tablet form.
- **Prednisone** is a synthetic hormone similar to hydrocortisone, a natural hormone produced by the adrenal glands. If your child has juvenile rheumatoid arthritis or another form

of painful arthritis, your doctor may prescribe prednisone, which is available as a syrup and a tablet.

- **Prednisolone** is available as syrup (Prelone) and a dissolvable tablet.

Possible Side Effects

Corticosteroids are associated with many side effects, including salt and fluid retention, high blood pressure, increased appetite, increased hair growth, increased production of acid in the stomach, increased sensitivity to the sun, and damage to the hip joints (aseptic necrosis of the hip). Long-term use of corticosteroids can result in acne, reduced wound healing, susceptibility to viral and fungal infections such as thrush, and eye problems (glaucoma). Because corticosteroids increase your child's susceptibility to illness, you will need to be especially careful to avoid exposure to viral diseases. If your child does come into contact with a sick child, call your child's doctor immediately. Also let your child's doctor know that he is taking corticosteroids before getting any immunizations or vaccinations.

Cortocosteroids are also associated with an increased risk of osteopenia (thinning and weakening of the structure of the bones) in children who take long courses of these drugs. This will lead to a susceptibility to bone fractures, especially compression fractures of the spine. According to a report presented at the Annual European Congress of Rheumatology in June 2003, the risk of bone fracture increased in children who received four or more courses of oral corticosteroids in the previous year. Because children who are in pain tend to exercise less, which also weakens the bones, it is important that you, your physician, and/or a physical therapist encourage your child to engage in regular weight-bearing activities (walking, tennis, jogging, volleyball, basketball) to help protect against osteopenia.

How To Take Corticosteroids

It's important that your child take corticosteroids exactly as the doctor prescribes them. For children younger than twelve years, the dose is determined based on the child's body weight. To help prevent stomach irritation, these drugs should be taken with food.

If your child experiences side effects, call your doctor immediately, but do not stop giving the medication without your doctor's permission. He or she will tell you how to gradually taper down the dosage. Abruptly stopping these drugs can cause nausea and vomiting, confusion, fever, headache, peeling skin, weight loss, and loss of appetite.

In children with cancer, corticosteroids are sometimes given intravenously or via injection if the child is hospitalized. If your child is not hospitalized, your doctor will prescribe a form most suitable for your child.

FAMOTIDINE AND PEPPERMINT OIL

Famotidine is a histamine H2 blocker used to treat peptic ulcers. In children with chronic pain, it is sometimes prescribed to treat recurrent abdominal pain (RAP), especially if the pain is thought to be partially related to reflux of stomach acids into the esophagus, known as gastroesophageal reflux disease (GERD). Peppermint oil, although not a drug, is also used to treat RAP that is associated with irritable bowel syndrome, a condition in which children experience pain associated with alternating bouts of constipation and diarrhea.

How Famotidine and Peppermint Oil Work

Famotidine has been approved by the Food and Drug Administration for use in infants, children, and teenagers. Famotidine blocks the activity of histamine (a substance the body produces naturally), which in turn reduces the secretion of hydrochloric acid in the stomach. Once the level of stomach hydrochloric acid is reduced, the stomach lining and esophagus can better heal themselves. Several studies show that famotidine is effective in children who have RAP and indigestion.

Peppermint oil capsules are powerful muscle relaxants that are widely used in England for irritable bowel syndrome and by some physicians in the United States. The capsules are specially coated (enteric-coated) to allow them to remain intact in the stomach and small intestines, then to release the peppermint oil in the colon and rectum, where they are most effective. Peppermint oil capsules have been shown to provide significant pain relief in children with irritable bowel syndrome.

How to Take Famotidine and Peppermint Oil

Carbonated drinks, citrus fruits and juices, and acidic foods and liquids, such as tomatoes and tomato juice, can interfere with the effectiveness of famotidine, so your child should avoid these foods and beverages while taking famotidine. Famotidine is available in tablets, powder for suspension, disintegrating tablets, and chewable tablets. The disintegrating tablets dissolve immediately in the mouth and don't require any water. To minimize the possibility of side effects, your child should take famotidine with food. Peppermint oil capsules should be taken between meals.

Possible Side Effects

Some of the side effects your child may experience while taking famotidine include constipation, diarrhea, dizziness, drowsiness, fatigue, headache, nausea, and vomiting. Peppermint oil capsules typically don't cause side effects, although rare cases of heartburn have been reported.

NONSTEROIDAL ANTIINFLAMMATORY DRUGS

Nonsteroidal antiinflammatory drugs (NSAIDs) are medications that reduce inflammation, swelling, fever, and joint stiffness and, in the process, also relieve pain.They do this by blocking the activity of an enzyme called cyclo-oxygenase, or COX. COX exists in at least two forms, COX-1 and COX-2 (there is a recently discovered COX-3, but its role and importance haven't yet been well defined by scientists). The COX-2 enzyme causes the inflammation associated with pain, while COX-1 is important for regulating the acidity of the stomach and the function of the blood cells that help blood to clot, among other things. The older over-the-counter NSAIDs on the market block the "good" COX-1 as well as COX-2, and thus produce more side effects, while the newer NSAIDs that are available by prescription only are selective COX-2 blockers.

NSAIDs are considered to be relatively safe and effective in treating many types of chronic pain in children. In fact, NSAIDs are probably prescribed for children more than any other type of painkiller.

Conditions Treated with Nonsteroidal Antiinflammatory Drugs

- Back pain
- Complex regional pain syndrome
- Chronic daily headache
- Facial pain
- Fibromyalgia
- Juvenile rheumatoid arthritis and other less common arthritic conditions that affect children (e.g., systemic lupus erythematosus, ankylosing spondylitis, Reiter's syndrome, dermatomyositis)
- Migraine

Types of Nonsteroidal Antiinflammatory Drugs

There are several types of NSAIDS, some of which are available over the counter, others by prescription only, and some in both forms. Of the more than one dozen NSAIDs on the market, the Food and Drug Administration has approved aspirin, ibuprofen, naproxen, and tolmetin sodium for children. The first three are available over the counter and by prescription, and the latter is by prescription only. Doctors can prescribe any of the unapproved NSAIDs for children, however, if the approved drugs do not effectively control symptoms.

- **Aspirin.** Aspirin should *not* be given to children younger than fifteen years because of the risk of Reye's syndrome. This syndrome can develop in children who take aspirin who are also suffering with a viral infection, especially influenza or chicken pox. Yes, I know there are children's aspirin brands on the market, but why take the risk of your child getting this often fatal disease when there are much safer medications he or she can take?
- **Ibuprofen** (Advil, Motrin, Nuprin) is available in chewable tablets and liquid forms.
- **Naproxen** (Naproxyn, Aleve) comes in tablets and liquid. Its advantage is that it need be given only twice a day, but unfortunately the liquid form doesn't taste as good to children as liquid ibuprofen.
- **Tolmetin** (Tolectin) is available in tablets and capsules.
- **COX-2 inhibitors** (celecoxib [Celebrex], valdecoxib [Bextra], and rofecoxib [Vioxx]) are among the newest NSAIDs on the market. They are associated with a lower risk of gastrointestinal side effects than the other, older NSAIDs. COX-2 inhibitors are particularly effective in treating chronic pain because they have a selective action within the spinal cord inhibiting COX-2, while the nonselective COX inhibitors do not have this effect. Another advantage of the COX-2 agents is that they have no effect on blood clotting, an important

consideration in some patients. However, it is important to note that none of the COX-2 inhibitors has been approved for use in children. Additionally, rofecoixib (Vioxx) was removed from the market in September 2004 by its manufacturer because of a significantly increased risk of cardiovascular events such as heart attack and stroke, and recent studies are suggesting that celecoxib and valdecoxib may have similar dangerous side effects. The use of these COX-2 inhibitors to treat chronic pain in children is not recommended.

Possible Side Effects

The most common side effect of the nonselective COX NSAIDs is gastritis, irritation of the stomach lining. This irritation can progress and cause bleeding or ulcers. Symptoms of gastritis include stomach pain, nausea, vomiting, poor appetite, or dark stools.

Some children who take NSAIDs bruise more easily or experience more nosebleeds than usual. This can occur because NSAIDs cause the blood to clot less easily than normal by inhibiting the small cells in the blood that initiate blood clotting, called platelets. This is usually not a major concern, but if your child is taking NSAIDS and needs to undergo surgery or tooth extraction, he or she should stop taking the drugs at least one week before the procedure to prevent excessive bleeding. This precaution also applies to children who have platelet disorders or to those receiving cancer chemotherapy. Make sure your health-care provider knows what medications your child is taking well before the procedure is to take place.

All the NSAIDs may have a bad effect on kidney function. This is generally not a problem in children, but children who already have a kidney problem should usually not receive any of the drugs in this class, not even the COX-2 inhibitors.

Other possible side effects from NSAIDs include liver irritation, which your doctor can monitor by taking regular blood tests; itchy rash; ringing in the ears (usually associated with aspirin use); and pseudoporphyria (development of blisters or scratches on the skin caused by sun exposure in fair-skinned, blue-eyed children; associated with naproxen use). If you notice your child has any of these or any other unusual symptoms, contact your doctor as soon as possible.

How to Take Nonsteroidal Antiinflammatory Drugs

Different children respond in different ways to different NSAIDs. Therefore, your doctor may need to change your child's dose or type of medication several times before finding the one that works best for your child. This approach is common, so do not worry if the first drug your doctor tries doesn't provide all the relief you expected. You or someone in your child's pain management team should explain this to him or her as well (see Chapter 7).

Because NSAIDs can cause some stomach irritation, they should be taken immediately after your child has a meal or a snack. A glass of juice or a piece of fruit is sufficient for most children. Children should never take NSAIDs and acetaminophen at the same time.

OPIOIDS (NARCOTICS)

Opioids are potent pain-killing drugs that are used primarily for treatment of severe short-term or chronic pain. Because they are much stronger than their milder counterparts, they are also associated with more side effects. However, judicious use of opioids in children with chronic pain is usually very safe and can make a significant, positive difference in the life of a child who lives with pain.

Conditions Treated with Opioids

Although opioids are used to treat the following conditions in children, they typically are administered only after other measures have failed to provide sufficient relief.

- Cancer pain
- Complex regional pain syndrome (in some cases)
- Migraine (in some cases)
- Sickle cell anemia (sickle cell crises)

Types of Opioids

Each of the following opioids differs in how long their pain-killing actions last and how they should be taken. Because opioids have a high risk of side effects, you need to observe your child carefully when he or she is taking these drugs.

- **Codeine.** This drug is considered to be a mild opioid and is available as an oral solution. Codeine is most commonly available in a combination form with acetaminophen (Tylenol with codeine) as an elixir or tablet.
- **Hydromorphone** (Dilaudid). This strong opioid is available as liquid, tablet, rectal suppository, and injection.

- **Morphine** (MS-Contin, MS-Immediate Release, and others). Morphine is a strong opioid and is available in capsules and tablets (both regular and sustained-release), liquid, suppositories, and injection.
- **Oxycodone** (OxyIR, OxyContin). Another strong opioid, it is available as a capsule, tablet, liquid, and controlled release tablet. It is also combined with acetaminophen in drugs such as Percocet, Roxicet, and Tylox.
- **Fentanyl.** Fentanyl is most often used in a hospital setting as an injection, but recently has become available as a skin patch that slowly releases the drug through the skin and into the bloodstream (Duragesic), and also as a lozenge that can be sucked (Actiq), releasing the drug into the mouth where some is absorbed through the lining of the mouth and some is swallowed and absorbed in the stomach. Children who can't tolerate oral medications may be given the fentanyl patch or may use the lozenge effectively. The patches are not appropriate for short-term or acute pain, but are useful for long-term pain that is not progressing rapidly and that requires little dose adjustments over time. One patch is usually applied every forty-eight to seventy-two hours. It usually takes about twenty-four hours for the first patch that is applied to begin eliminating pain. After the first patch is used, pain relief is sustained without interruption when the patch is changed. Thus, children with severe pain who use a fentanyl patch need to take painkillers that provide immediate relief along with it after introduction of the patch for the first time.The fentanyl oral lozenge (Actiq) is not available in a small enough dose for small children, but can be effectively used by larger children and teenagers. Unlike

the patch, pain relief from the lozenge is very rapid, generally occurring in minutes. Thus the Actiq lozenge is effective for breakthrough pain. The Food and Drug Administration has approved use of the lozenge only for breakthrough cancer pain.

How Opioids Work

Opioids work on the brain and spinal cord and can change a person's perception of pain by interfering with the pain signals in these two areas of the body. The brain has naturally occurring pleasure sites that contains opioid receptors, which attract chemicals that turn on the pleasure system. The effect of an opioid depends on what kind of drug is given and how it's administered. The faster an opioid reaches the brain, the faster it provides relief and a pleasurable, dreamy feeling. Opioids that are given through an IV tube reach the brain much faster than a tablet or other oral dose does. After an opioid drug reaches the brain, activation by the drug of receptors in the brain causes the brain to send chemicals (norepinephrine) down to the spinal cord, that then interrupt the transmission of pain signals arriving from the body.

Side Effects

Constipation is one of the first and most troublesome side effects some children experience, usually after a few days, when they begin to take opioids. You can help avoid this complication by making sure your child drinks lots of water or other liquids and eats high-fiber foods, such as fresh vegetables and whole grains, rather than low-fiber foods such as white bread. If this isn't possible, you may ask your doctor for a stool softener, which will make it easier for your child to pass stool. You will need to take note of your child's bowel movements while he or she is taking opioids. If two or three days pass without a bowel movement, contact your doctor so a laxative can be recommended.

Other side effects some children experience within the first few days of starting opioids are nausea, itchiness (especially facial itchiness), difficulty urinating, dizziness, confusion, nightmares, and drowsiness. Some parents tell me that their children become grouchy, mean, or depressed while taking opioids. Unlike constipation, which generally persists as long as the opioid medication is taken, these other side effects usually wear off after a period of days, or sometimes weeks. If any of these symptoms persist, contact your doctor. He or she may change the dosage or prescribe a different opioid.

Lingering Myths about Opioid Use in Children

The most common question parents ask me about opioids is, "Won't my child become addicted to these drugs?" The simple answer is, no.

Patients, including infants, children, and adolescents, will become tolerant to taking opioids, and they will become physically dependent upon opioids if they are taken for more than a week or so. However, it is extremely important for you (and your child's pediatrician) to understand that this is not the same thing as being addicted to the opioid medication.

Here's the explanation of what happens when a child takes opioids for pain management. After she has been taking opioids for a few days, her body slowly begins to develop a physiological dependence on the drug. This means your child's body has become accustomed to having the drug in its system, and has made certain chemical changes in itself because the drug is there. Thus if the drug is abruptly stopped, the body will feel ill not having this chemical it has become accustomed to having. That is, the body has become *physically* dependent on the drug, but *not* psychologically addicted. The other thing that slowly happens as the body becomes accustomed to having the opioid in its system is that it develops *tolerance* to the medicine. This means that over time, the same dose will produce less and less of an effect, and therefore the dose will slowly need to be increased to produce the desired degree of pain relief. These phenomena of physical dependence and tolerance nearly always occur together, and indeed probably have the same biochemical mechanism.

By the way, this is something that is not unique to opioids; it also occurs with many other medications that are commonly prescribed, such as corticosteroids or inhalers for asthma, insulin for diabetes, and so on, yet we don't refer to our children with asthma as being "addicted" to their inhalers, or our diabetic children as being "addicted" to their insulin. Unfortunately in our society, opioid medication is stigmatized because of the propensity of a small minority of people to use the drug recreationally and illegally, and this stigma sometimes gets in the way of providing effective pain relief to those who need and deserve it most.

Remember, physical dependence and tolerance are not the same thing as an addiction. Addiction is a genetically based psychiatric disease that is characterized by drug craving, using the drug for nonmedicinal purposes, and using the drug in a self-destructive manner. Addiction is usually seen in connection with lying, stealing, or other dishonest or illegal behaviors. Addiction specialists estimate that approximately 5 percent of the American population have the genetic basis for becoming addicted *given the right social circumstances.* The other 95 percent are not at risk for addiction, even if given strong medications such as opioids. Indeed, even those in the minority 5 percent who are at risk for addiction will usually not develop addiction behaviors if given opioids for a therapeutic purpose.

Use of opioids allows your child to live as active and pain-free a life as possible. When your child no longer needs the drug to control the pain, your doctor should gradually decrease the dose over a period of days or weeks to prevent your child from experiencing withdrawal symptoms, which include diarrhea, cramps, trembling, sweating, insomnia, and irritability.

Another question parents ask is, "What happens if the opioid stops working?" Every child is different, and sometimes it is necessary to change the pain medication if one is no longer effective. When the body gets used to a drug and the drug doesn't provide the pain relief it did originally, this is called *tolerance.* Your doctor can then increase the dose or add another drug to the treatment plan that will enhance the effect of the opioid.

Sometimes parents of children who have cancer worry when their doctor prescribes an opioid because they think this means their child is going to die. In fact, opioids can be prescribed at any time during the course of cancer and it does not mean the child is going to die. Opioids are also prescribed for severe chronic non-cancer pain, such as experienced by children with severe arthritis, CRPS, sickle cell disease, and the like.

When a doctor orders an opioid for a child who has cancer, it means he or she has found a drug that will allow the child to get relief from pain and still function in as normal a manner as possible.

A Final Word About Opioid Prescriptions

The writing of opioid prescriptions and the dispensing of opioids by pharmacies are tightly controlled and monitored by state governments. Because of this, and because opioids have a street value if they are diverted from the patient, many physicians are reluctant or even paranoid about prescribing them. The fact is that physicians must be very careful about prescribing opioids and keep careful track of their use. Many physicians' offices require patients and/or their families to sign a "contract" describing the mutual responsibilities of doctor and patient when opioids are prescribed, and describe what will happen if a patient takes more than prescribed, loses the prescription or the medicine, or has the medicine stolen. If your child's regular doctor or pain doctor wishes you to sign such a contract, don't feel that they are being suspicious or antagonistic. It is a routine practice in many places, designed to protect both doctor and patient and satisfy state regulatory requirements.

TRIPTANS

Triptan medications mimic naturally occurring brain serotonin, and thus affect the serotonin receptors in the brain and constrict

MANAGING PAIN MEDICATIONS AT HOME

If your child is taking pain medication, you should know the answers to the following questions. Don't leave your doctor's office until you do! The answers may differ depending on your child's condition and the medications he or she is taking.

- What should I do if my child forgets to take a scheduled dose of his/her medication?
- What should I do if my child's pain returns before it's time for him/her to take the next scheduled dose?
- Am I allowed to increase the dose of my child's pain medication without calling the doctor?
- What should I do if my child wakes up in pain in the middle of the night?

blood vessels. These drugs typically can relieve pain within minutes to two hours of taking them, depending upon the drug and the route of administration.

Conditions Treated with Triptans

Triptans are used to treat migraine and other severe headache.

Types of Triptans

Triptans are available as several different medications. Even though they all work in a similar way, some may work better and faster for your child than others, and your child may have fewer or milder side effects with some than others. Also, talk to your doctor about how often your child should take triptans. If they are taken too frequently, they can cause rebound headache—head pain that is actually caused by the very medications taken to control it.

- **Sumatriptan.** The first triptan to reach the market was sumatriptan (Imitrex). It is available as a pill, nasal spray, and a subcutaneous injection. The nasal spray is convenient and easy to use for children and the form I often prescribe for them, although it is very bitter tasting. The fastest relief from migraine headaches occurs with sumatriptan injection, but few children choose to take a medication by injection even though the pain relief is much faster and more complete.
- **Naratriptan.** Naratriptan (Amerge) is available in pill form, and is roughly equivalent to sumatriptan in its effectiveness.
- **Rizatriptan.** Under the brand name Maxalt, this triptan is available in pills that can be swallowed or pills that are allowed to melt in the mouth. This latter form is helpful for children who have difficulty swallowing pills, or when vomiting complicates migraine headaches. Rizatriptan is also superior to sumatriptan pills in effectiveness.
- **Zolmitriptan.** Zomig is available in nasal spray, pill, and dissolvable pill forms, the latter a form that melts in the mouth and doesn't need to be swallowed. Studies have generally shown Zomig nasal spray to be superior to sumatriptan, and to be the fastest noninjection drug for headache relief.
- **Other triptans.** Almotriptan (Axert), eletriptan (Relpax), and frovatriptan (Frova) are more recently approved triptans

that work in the same way as those listed above. They are available only as pills that must be swallowed.

How to Choose a Triptan

There are now nearly ten triptans on the market, and choosing between them may seem confusing. None are yet available as inexpensive generic drugs, so they are all quite expensive if you are paying out of pocket. None are "approved" for use in children under eighteen years of age, but all are safe and effective in children.

Because there is not a major difference in the effectiveness among these drugs, the first thing to do is to check to see which of these medications have been approved for reimbursement by your insurance company. After that, I recommend you choose based upon how they are administered, in other words, by pill, oral dissolvable tablet, nasal spray, or injection. The injectable form of Imitrex is certainly the most rapidly effective form available, but it is the rare child who will go along with an uncomfortable shot in the arm or leg, even with the promise of relieving an agonizing headache (by the way, it's not just the needle that hurts, but the sumatriptan itself stings when injected). But it's hard to argue with relief that occurs in minutes rather than an hour or more.

The nasal sprays (Imitrex and Zomig) are the second most rapid way to relieve a migraine, and are a good choice for those children who cannot swallow pills, or who vomit when they have a migraine.

Finally, I prefer the oral dissolvable tablets (Maxalt and Zomig) for other cases, again because of the problem with nausea and vomiting that accompanies most migraines. These dissolvable tablets are how I treat my own migraines and those in my own children.

Few studies have done (if you'll pardon the expression) head-to-head comparisons of effectiveness of these drugs to help us choose among them. The typical way these drugs are evaluated is to look at the percentage of migraine sufferers whose headaches improve to mild or better two hours after taking the medicine. Typically, 20 to 40 percent of those patients who take an inert pill (a placebo) will have this kind of relief, and 50 to 60 percent of those with migraine will have this amount of improvement after a triptan. As you can see, as good as the triptans are they are not magic bullets for migraine headaches.

When many smaller experiments are put together and statistically analyzed as a group (this is called a meta-analysis), rizatriptan (Maxalt) seems to perform slightly better than the other drugs. However, the data reported to the FDA by the manufacturer of eletriptan (Relpax) show still better rates of improvement with their highest dose (55 to 77 percent) than other drugs typically show.

Side Effects

All of the triptans can cause similar side effects, including nausea, dizziness, sleepiness, and a feeling of burning or tightening of the neck, chest, and face. In most cases, however, these side effects are mild. Use of the nasal spray can cause nasal dryness and a bitter taste in the mouth, something that may not be well tolerated by children whose migraines are complicated by nausea. Because all the triptans cause constriction of blood vessels, they should be avoided in anybody with coronary artery disease (thankfully rare in children), but also in children with a rare form of migraine that affects the brainstem, called basilar migraine, and in children with another rare migraine variant called hemiplegic migraine.

How to Use Triptans

The triptans can be taken with or without food and should be used at the very first indication of a migraine. The earlier a triptan is taken during a migraine headache, the more effective it will be. They are not for treatment of everyday headache. If the headache does not get better in two hours, or improves but comes back in two hours or more, a second dose may be taken. Generally no more than two doses in twenty-four hours should be taken.

EXTRA-SPECIAL DRUG DELIVERY

For many children, their pain medications come in the form of a pill, syrup, or liquid they can take at home. Sometimes, however, children need to be hospitalized for pain control when other efforts have not been successful, and physicians then often turn to more potent or invasive pain-relief methods. We talk about four here.

Epidural Catheter

One excellent pain control method for hospitalized children is use of an epidural or spinal catheter. In this approach, a catheter (a tiny, narrow tube) is placed within the spine, just outside of the fluid-filled spinal canal, and near the spinal cord where the pain signals are coming in from the body and being transmitted to the brain. The catheter delivers pain mediation into a space between the spine's protective cover (the dura) and the spinal column. This type of nerve block is perhaps familiar to most people as the type used to help expectant moms during childbirth. One advantage of an epidural catheter is that the medications are administered at doses that are only one-tenth or even one one-hundredth of the dose that would be needed conventionally, because it is being delivered directly to the nerves. This means your child is less likely to experience the side effects associated with the drug used.

If your child needs an epidural catheter, the doctor will first apply a topical anesthetic to the skin to numb the area where the catheter will be inserted. Sometimes I place epidural catheters in children who are heavily sedated or even under anesthesia, so that they experience no discomfort or memory of its placement. Once the catheter is in place, the chosen medications can be injected. An epidural catheter also does not interfere with your child's ability to walk. One side effect of a catheter, however, may be some numbness or even weakness in the legs. Catheters can be left in place for a few days, a few weeks using a slightly different technique for their placement, or may even be permanently implanted if your child needs chronic pain management at home for a long time.

Patient Controlled Analgesia

Another method used by some hospitalized children is PCA—patient controlled analgesia. This approach can be used with an

IV line or an epidural catheter. The PCA allows a child to push a button on a small device, which signals a computer-controlled pump to deliver a predetermined amount of medication through the IV line or catheter. Thus the child can decide when he needs more pain medication. Children as young as six or seven can use a PCA pump independently.

There are safety mechanisms built into PCA to prevent toxicity or overdosage. For example, the computer is programmed with maximum doses, doses are spaced out in time to allow a previous dose's full effect to be felt before another one is administered (even if the button continues to be pushed), and finally and most importantly, if a child begins to get too high a dose, he will simply doze off and stop pushing the button, thus stopping the delivery of more medicine.

Tara is a ten-year-old girl with cystic fibrosis who came to the hospital for a liver transplant. After her surgery, she was in the intensive care unit for two days, and then moved to a regular room on the third day. To manage her pain, she was given a bolus dose (a concentrated dose of a drug given intravenously) of fentanyl every two hours. Unfortunately, this dose only provided about twenty minutes of satisfactory pain relief, and then 100 minutes of pain until she could receive her next bolus dose. In fact, once the fentanyl wore off, Tara reported pain at 9 to 10 out of 10 on a pain scale. She didn't want to eat and she couldn't sleep. Unfortunately, this scenario is not uncommon, as many children (and adults) who need pain medication are undermedicated, and so they spend the time in between doses watching the clock, waiting for the nurse to bring them relief.

At that point, Tara's surgeons asked us to manage her pain. We immediately put her on a continuous low-dose infusion of hydromorphone (we chose hydromorphone because it lasts longer than fentanyl) via a pump and also gave her the same drug by PCA. While the pump provided a continuous low level of medication while she slept at night and took naps during the day, she also now had the option to push the button for additional medication when the pump wasn't enough. This is important because when children fall asleep and they are using PCA only, they will not get any doses during sleep and will wake up in pain. Because PCA delivers only small doses, it takes too long for the low doses to provide adequate relief when the pain returns. Thus using both the pump and PCA provides continuous relief.

Once Tara was on the pump and PCA, her pain scores dropped to less than 4, she was able to sleep and eat, and she also felt well enough to play card games with her mother and sister. After about eight days, we tapered her off the PCA and pump, she was given oral painkillers, and then sent home.

There has been some controversy about the safety of using continuous infusions of medications. Although there have been some problems with background infusions in adults, safety studies in children have shown that it is as safe as PCA alone and that there are fewer side effects than using PCA alone provided the background infusion dose is very low.

I routinely see children as young as four years old use PCA with some parental or nursing assistance, which means the parents or nurses talk with the child and then they decide jointly whether the pain is severe enough to push the button. It's important that the child be allowed to push the button, and not the parents or the nurse. This gives the child a sense of control over his or her pain. Whether a child pushes the button after talking with parents or nurses or is old enough to do so on her own, parents should know that the system is designed so children cannot give themselves an overdose of medication.

PCA may also be used for children who because of injury, surgery, or disability lack the ability to press the button. In those cases, a parent may push the button for them, but only when told to do so by the child. This keeps the child in control, and preserves the safety mechanism of preventing children from receiving more opioid than they need.

Nerve Blocks

A nerve block involves injecting medication, most often a local anesthetic, into a specific area to relieve pain that is coming from a specific nerve. You are probably familiar with nerve blocks if you've ever had dental work done with local anesthesia. If you have experienced such a nerve block, you know how effective they can be.

Because children, especially younger ones, are not fond of needles, I find the best approach is to place a catheter to deliver the nerve block, rather than give several single injections at intervals of days to weeks. The catheter is then infused continuously, for two or three weeks more or less, using an external pump that contains the needed medication, be it a local anesthetic such as lidocaine, or steroids to help reduce inflammation.

Continuously blocking the nerves to a painful part of the body affected by either somatic pain (for example, after an injury to a leg) or neuropathic pain (for example, in children with CRPS or with phantom pain after an amputation) often allows the sensitized nervous system to cool off, resulting in prolonged pain relief or more easily controlled milder pain after the catheter is removed and the local anesthetics wear off.

Nerve blocks are not a cure-all, and they do not provide permanent relief. However, they do allow the highly stressed nervous system to relax and help it to regain its normal function. This is especially important because it allows patients to participate in critically needed physical therapy, as was the case with Barbara, whom I'll describe below.

Sympathetic Nerve Block

Sympathetic nerve blocks are different from peripheral nerve blocks, because they are designed to numb only the sympathetic nerves, not the nerves that carry sensation or the nerves that control muscle movement. Sympathetic nerve blocks are used specifically for the management of the pain of CRPS.

The sympathetic nerves are located right next to the spinal column, and can be blocked in the neck if CRPS affects an arm, or in the low back if CRPS affects a leg or foot. I usually have to perform these blocks under deep sedation or general anesthesia, because they are generally uncomfortable for most children, and it is actually safer to have a still and quiet child than one who is uncomfortable and squirmy while inserting the block needle.

One day, sixteen-year-old Barbara was chasing her dog in the yard when she slipped on the grass and smacked her hand against a stone wall as she fell. She developed tendonitis in the hand, which over the next month or two developed into CRPS. Her hand was constantly painful, and she was unable to move

HELPING THE MEDICINE GO DOWN

Many medications are available in liquid form, which can make them easier to give or for the child to take him or herself. However, these medicines don't always taste great. Here are a few tips on how to get your child to take medicine that may have an undesirable taste.

- Mix the medicine into some food. Sweet foods, such as sweetened applesauce or pudding, are often good at camouflaging a foul-tasting drug. Use a small amount of food that you know the child will eat, or else he or she will not get the entire dose.
- Have your child hold his or her nose when taking the drug. Taste is dulled when you can't smell what you're ingesting.
- Have your child eat or suck on something very cold (e.g., an ice pop, sherbet, an ice cube) immediately before taking the medicine. The cold will help numb the taste buds.
- Refrigerate the medicine (unless the drug specifically should not be kept cold). Some medicines taste better when they are cold.
- Have your child take the medicine through a straw that is placed far back into the mouth (but not enough to choke the child). This is an attempt to bypass the taste buds.

Remember: if the medication has a dropper or a medicine cup, use these to measure out the proper dose. Do **not** use a kitchen spoon, as they come in different sizes and you run the risk of giving your child either too little or too much medication.

her fingers out of a clenched position without experiencing severe pain. Her parents took her to an anesthesiologist, who performed a sympathetic nerve block. This procedure allowed her to immediately start physical and occupational therapy, but her pain relief was only temporary, so another nerve block was done one month after the first. Her doctor prescribed Neurontin and an antidepressant to help control the pain, but she discontinued both medications because of side effects, including headache, nausea, and sleepiness. These side effects were especially troublesome to Barbara, because they made it difficult for her to do well in school, which she enjoyed immensely and where she was an "A" student with her eye on Ivy League colleges.

Discouraged by the failure of her previous treatment, Barbara and her parents came to my clinic ten months after the incident in their yard. Barbara's hand was in a fist, and her hand was extremely painful to touch. We decided to hospitalize her so we could do a sympathetic block catheter in her neck, and she responded very well—her hand became warm and pink, and with aggressive physical and occupational therapy over the next four weeks, she was able to open her hand completely and hold and write with a pen. Once she left the hospital, she continued with therapy and relearned how to use her hand. Because CRPS can be a recurrent disease, she eventually needed another sympathetic block catheter many months later, but she was eventually able to regain full use of her hand.

BOTTOM LINE

Although medications are not typically my first line of defense against chronic pain, sometimes they are needed, even if for just a short time. This is especially true when I prescribe drugs so children can participate in intensive physical therapy that will help them regain control of affected limbs. Medications also become necessary when children would be otherwise incapacitated without them. Drugs alone are not the answer to chronic pain; various mind-body options that we discussed in previous chapters should be the basis of the pain-control approach you take for your child. However, we are fortunate in having a variety of safe and effective medications also at our disposal to complement the nonpharmaceutical approaches.

Chapter 7

KEEPING YOUR FAMILY HEALTHY

When a child experiences chronic pain, it's a family affair: parents, siblings, and sometimes even grandparents and other close relatives, all are part of the family dynamics. Although the child is the one who experiences the physical pain, those around him or her usually feel emotional stress, and often social and financial stress as well. Stress plays a large and critically important role in those dynamics and can determine how each family member relates to the hurting child and to each other. Stress and how well it is managed—or not managed—impacts the health of the child in chronic pain as well as the well-being of the family unit as a whole.

Living with a child who has chronic pain can cause family members to feel a range of emotions, including fear, anger, anxiety, helplessness, and shame. The energy from these emotions has an impact on each and every family member, and it can be very detrimental to both the hurting child and the other family members. If these emotions can be identified, understood, and managed; if family members can learn constructive ways to cope with the stress; and if parents can identify how they may be unconsciously contributing to their child's chronic pain, then the entire family unit can be healthier. Helping a child who has chronic pain is not just about healing the child; it's about healing the family members as well.

In this chapter we talk about the emotional roller coaster family members often ride when dealing with a child in chronic pain. We discuss how parents can be active participants in reducing their own stress and that of their child and in managing harmful emotions.

RIDING THE EMOTIONAL ROLLER COASTER

Your goal as a parent is to bring as much balance and normalcy to your child's life as you can. Perhaps that doesn't seem possible at the moment. Maybe the entire family's activities revolve around the child in chronic pain. Do you have to change appointments, cancel dinner plans, or miss work to take care of your child? Do you have other children who are struggling to understand why their brother or sister seems to be "different" or gets "special" attention? Have you had to change vacation plans or ask your other children to change their plans? All of these things and more can cause a great deal of emotional turmoil in a family.

"I love my child dearly," said Pamela, who clearly looked tense as she eased herself into a chair in my office. "I just never imagined I would be giving up so much of my life to meet his needs." Pamela's sentiments are echoed by many parents, some out loud, some silently to themselves. There isn't a lot of research on the impact of stress on parents of children who have chronic pain, but what little there is, and what my experience and that of my colleagues shows, is that the impact can be great.

First, consider some of the things that contribute to high stress in families who have a child in chronic pain. One of parents' biggest fears is the lack of a clear diagnosis or fear that a diagnosis was missed (see "The Missed Diagnosis" later in this chapter). Other factors that raise stress levels and set parents on an emotional roller coaster are frustration over the lack of simple treatment solutions and feelings of helplessness, of feeling unable to help their child.

Now take these feelings of frustration, helplessness, fear, and anxiety and think about all the areas of your life that can be affected when a child has chronic pain. One is the relationship between yourself and your child. You worry about your child, you get anxious when he or she is suffering; you may feel helpless or afraid. Your child senses these emotions and has anxieties of his or her own. Nerves can wear thin, and the stress and tension can take over your life. That's when we get parents like Pamela, who find themselves in emotional turmoil.

Sometimes the relationship between a child and parent—typically the mother—becomes emotionally unhealthy, where the mother and her child become overly emotionally dependent on each other, or they become best friends instead of maintaining a parent-child relationship. We call this "enmeshment." This type of emotional roller coaster can not only contribute to the child's pain but also prevent her from establishing a healthy, mature detachment and independence from the parent as the child enters adolescence. Such was the case with Karla.

Karla's Story

Donna took Karla, her twelve-year-old daughter, to their pediatrician after she complained about having a daily headache and stomach pain. Both types of pain started near the beginning of the school year (which is when many such pain complaints begin for children), and Karla remembers that the first time the pains appeared was after a fire drill at school. Following that incident, she began to have daily headaches that varied in location—sometimes on one side of her head, sometimes in the back, sometimes both sides—but they were always severe and throbbing and were accompanied by moderate to severe pain around her belly button. She also had an aversion to sound and sometimes experienced nausea and vomiting.

The pediatrician noted the symptoms, learned that both Donna and her mother had a history of migraine, and referred Karla to a neurologist, who performed a spinal tap, which was negative for any disease. He then started her on a program of valproic acid one month after her symptoms first appeared. She continued to take the medication for seven weeks, but it didn't provide any relief. The neurologist also tried Diamox, but it too was ineffective.

Karla was then referred to our clinic for nondrug management, and I saw her in February. It was apparent during her first visit that Karla and her mother were "best friends," and that Donna was, with good intentions, doing things that were actually detrimental to her daughter's recovery. In the beginning of the school year she would leave work and take Karla out of school at the drop of a hat, then spend the remainder of the day together with her. I outlined a treatment program for Karla that included new medications (nortriptyline for migraine prevention and sumatriptan nasal spray to stop episodes), biofeedback sessions, and psychotherapy, and Donna agreed.

We learned that Donna had given up her full-time job to cater to Karla's headaches, and often she would remove her daughter from school and take her home. Karla was missing three to four days of school per week, and since she declared that she "really didn't like school much," she didn't care. When she stayed home from school, her mother would prepare special meals for her or let her sleep or watch videos. Karla didn't have many friends at school, and soon her mother began to fulfill that role instead of her classmates.

This isn't to say that Karla didn't have headaches, or was fabricating her headaches. She (and her mother) both clearly had migraine. But what became clear was that even if Karla had a minor nagging headache, instead of simply coping, and carrying on with her day like most of us would do, she subconsciously learned that making the presence of that headache known resulted in lots of pleasurable things, like leaving school, hanging with Mom, and playing on the computer in her room. This kind of thing is called "secondary gain," which means when someone has something to gain in compensation for something that is undesirable. It is very important to nip secondary gain in the bud, because it can have an enormous impact on the ability of a child to learn appropriate coping strategies for dealing with pain.

After taking nortriptyline and sumatriptan and practicing biofeedback for several months, Karla was missing only a few days of school out of six weeks. I had asked her to keep a pain diary, and she noted that she had minor headaches three to four times a week, but only two severely incapacitating headaches during a six-week period, which she had successfully stopped with sumatriptan. It was interesting to note, however, that the positive response Karla experienced happened toward the end of the school year.

Karla continued to take the same medications during the summer and still kept her daily pain diary. Throughout the summer, she experienced only one minor attack, which she stopped with sumatriptan. Then when school started in September, she immediately reported a headache. On the second day of school, she wrote that she had a headache that was "3 to 4 out of 10." During the weekend, she didn't have a headache, but by Tuesday she had developed stomach pain after school. On Wednesday she had a headache, and then reported that she woke up at three in the morning with a headache on Thursday.

This pattern continued, with her reporting three to five headaches per week throughout September and October. I had increased her dose of nortriptyline near the beginning of the school year, and she asked to stop biofeedback because it wasn't helping. She did, however, agree to continue with psychotherapy. When the frequent headaches continued into November, I tapered her off nortriptyline and started propranolol and also switched to DHE nasal spray instead of the sumatriptan.

Although it was obvious that Karla's headaches and stomach pain were associated with stress at school as well as secondary gain, both Karla and her mother refused to accept that relationship. They also didn't understand the role that stress and behavior had in causing the headaches and that stress management and changes in behavior could provide relief. One good thing that did come out of the psychotherapy sessions is that Donna returned to full-time employment and no longer catered to her daughter's demands to stay home from school or to come home once a headache started. Even though Karla continued to have chronic daily headache and frequent migraines, she missed very little school.

By January, the propranolol hadn't produced any significant results, so I tapered her off the drug and started her on gabapentin. She agreed to try acupuncture, but stopped after a few sessions without results. For the rest of the school year, the summer, and into the next school year, she continued on daily gabapentin and DHE when needed, and the frequency and severity of her headaches decreased.

When Karla learned that her mother was going to have surgery in November, her headaches escalated dramatically. Faced with the fact that her mother wouldn't be at home for a week and would need time to recover once she returned home, Karla began to experience severe chronic daily headaches again and missed school nearly every day. She refused to talk to the psychologist any longer, and by January, Donna reported that Karla was out of control; that she threw tantrums, constantly told her mother to quit her job and stay home with her, and was completely frustrated and angry all the time. I recommended that she be hospitalized for behavior modification and pain rehabilitation, but Karla refused and Donna wouldn't make her go.

Because the psychologist couldn't speak directly with Karla, the alternative was for the psychologist to start a behavioral modification program through Donna. He and Donna set up strict limits around Karla's behavior, including helping with chores around the house and doing her homework before she could use her computer, with positive reinforcement when she behaved appropriately (e.g., phone privileges, get a favorite CD) and consequences when she did not (no phone privileges, no computer time). Donna put the limits into play for the rest of the school year, but with limited success.

During the summer, Karla developed trichotillomania, a form of obsessive-compulsive disorder in which individuals (usually girls) pull out their hair. Within a few months Karla was virtually bald, and she and her mother finally acknowledged that Karla had an emotional disorder and agreed to see a psychiatrist. He started her on paroxatine (Paxil) and psychotherapy. Karla continues to have migraines and to take Paxil, and now Topamax. But her attendance and performance at school have been good, her migraine headaches are much reduced in frequency, small nonmigraine headaches no longer take her out of school, and happily the trichotillomania is under control with the help of Paxil and support groups and her hair is regrowing.

Karla's situation demonstrates how there can be many factors that can contribute to or have an underlying role in a child's chronic pain. Along with the strong family history of migraine, Karla also had significant stress associated with going to school and clearly had an inappropriate relationship with her mother. The appearance of her obsessive-compulsive behavior—trichotillomania—was, along with her migraines, a way she demonstrated her inability to handle stress. When she did practice coping skills, her head pain improved and her school attendance was better. However, she continually refused to cooperate with her psychologist and with her mother, and this made treatment more difficult. If she had been more willing to work on her coping and stress management skills, we would have been able to rely less on medications to manage her migraines. However, it can be difficult to help a twelve-year-old understand the relationship between mental and physical health. Our hope is that if Karla keeps seeing her psychologist as she matures, she, along with her mother's help, will realize that she can have much more control over her migraines and her obsessive-compulsive behavior if she practices coping skills.

Other Emotional Issues

One significant emotional issue is the relationship between the child in pain and his or her siblings. Otherwise healthy brothers and sisters may resent any additional attention or special privileges the child in pain gets, or they may feel embarrassed that something is wrong with their sibling. Others get angry at the hurting child and are cruel, emotionally and/or physically. These are emotions that must be dealt with in a professional and loving way.

Child psychologists can be instrumental in helping parents recognize the need for them to pay attention to the feelings of siblings of children who have chronic pain and how to balance the time they spend with all of their children. Usually this understanding can be achieved after just one or two meetings between the psychologist and the parents, who are given some ways that are specific to their situation on how to handle any hurt or angry feelings their other children may be feeling. Generally, those ways include having parents shift from reinforcing the pain behavior of the child in pain to reinforcing adaptive behavior, and also spending more time with their other children.

For example, ten-year-old Leeann used to clear the table and load the dishwasher every night after dinner. When her CRPS confined her to a wheelchair or to walking with crutches, she whined and said she couldn't do her chores any more. Clearing the table and loading the dishwasher then fell to her nine-year-old sister, Jessica, who was still expected to water the garden every other night. Jessica began to bully her older sister, and said to her parents, "why should I be punished just because she's sick?" Over a period of about two months, Jessica transformed from being a loving, happy child into an angry and defiant one as she saw her parents catering to Leeann's needs.

The girls' parents, Marie and George, became concerned with Jessica's behavior and mentioned it to the child psychologist Leeann was seeing. He asked Marie and George when they first noticed the change in behavior and what they thought had precipitated it. He then asked them to list all the ways normal family life had changed since Leeann had been diagnosed with CRPS. One major thing they admitted was that they were not able to go out as a family as much as they used to. While they used to go see a movie every few weeks, they now stayed home and rented a video, usually one that Leeann wanted to see. They also talked about how Jessica had taken over Leeann's chores, and that their younger daughter was clearly angry with her sister.

"I feel like I'm walking on eggs with my daughters," said Marie. "They fight all the time, and Jessica can say very cruel things. Then Leeann cries, and I have to comfort her, and then Jessica accuses me of always being on Leeann's side. Our family life has become a battleground."

The psychologist explained how Marie and George were reinforcing Leeann's pain behavior by catering to her and allowing her to get away with not doing chores. He pointed out that even if it took Leeann longer to do the chores she used to do or she was slower doing new chores, it was important that she share responsibilities, just like her younger sister did.

Marie and George then sat down with their daughters and explained that the chores would be evenly divided between them; that they could either switch between their two chores every month, or each could continue to do the same chore all the time, the choice would be up to them. The girls decided they wanted to switch every month, although Leeann complained that she couldn't load the dishwasher from her wheelchair. Marie helped Leeann practice taking dishes from the dining room to the dishwasher in her wheelchair, and Leeann soon felt comfortable doing this chore. Marie and George also have been taking the girls out to the movies, even though Leeann usually needs her crutches, and they make sure they allow Jessica to choose the movie half the time.

I cannot stress enough that in most families with children with chronic pain, it is of great importance not to allow the establishment of patterns of disability behavior. This is much easier said than done, because our natural instinct as parents is to shelter and isolate children who are ill.

Depression

It has been well established that children (and adults) who have chronic pain often also experience depression and anxiety, and that these emotional states can have a significant impact on pain severity and the effectiveness of any therapy and rehabilitation efforts. According to a recent study (April 2004), children with chronic abdominal pain are considerably more likely to have a psychiatric diagnosis of anxiety or depressive disorder. The study's researchers note that about 80 percent of children in the study who had chronic abdominal pain had an anxiety disorder and that about 40 percent also had depression.

Sometimes depression or other emotional disorders are

caused by the same thing that causes the chronic pain problem. We know, for example, that migraine headaches are significantly associated with a tendency toward depression, and also toward obsessive-compulsive behavior disorders (just as in Karla's case above), but not other psychiatric conditions. This doesn't mean that all children with migraine have these problems; indeed they don't. But the genes that lead a person to be a migraine sufferer are closely related or linked to the genes that cause some forms of depression or obsessive-compulsive disorder, and the two conditions therefore often coexist.

In other cases, depression is caused by chronic pain, and what could be more obvious than that? If a condition hurts and stops your child from doing the things she wants to do, and makes her feel "different," it's no wonder that feelings of sadness and low self-esteem soon follow.

The fact that chronic pain and depression and/or anxiety are intricately entwined means we need to treat these disorders as part of a child's therapy for chronic pain. Yet all too often, children in chronic pain are treated by pediatricians or general practitioners who are not trained to take a holistic view of chronic pain; that is, a mind-body approach. The result is that depression and anxiety go unrecognized and thus untreated in these children.

Chronic pain is a complex condition that requires a multifaceted approach, and that includes attention to psychiatric issues. This is a point that is sometimes difficult for parents to understand or accept, because they often feel that if their child (or if they) are referred to a psychologist, psychiatrist, or other mental health professional, there is something "wrong" with their child's mind or that their child is mentally ill, or that we are suggesting that their pain is "in their head." As you will see in the section entitled "Psychotherapy: A Critical Element," this is not true at all.

Financial Stress

Living with a child who has chronic pain also can be a financial strain on a family. Even if a family has insurance, some medications and procedures may not be covered and so families have to pay for them out of pocket. Some working parents miss lots of work or even lose or quit their jobs to care for their hurting child. Given the large number of single-parent families today, this can be a tremendous burden on some parents.

Has your whole family been ready to go on a trip or attend an event, when the child with chronic pain suddenly became too ill to go? How did your other children feel about it? How did you feel? And, equally important, how did the child in pain feel? Did he or she feel responsible for ruining everyone's day? Did he or she feel like a bad person?

The emotional roller coaster that children in pain and their families experience can be just as devastating as the physical pain. Clearly, in many cases, as we've seen especially with CRPS, and recurrent abdominal pain and migraine as well, emotional stress and anxieties are directly associated with the manifestation of pain. I have seen patients with CRPS who had pink, warm, nonpainful hands or feet one minute, and within minutes of hearing stressful news or being faced with an emotional situation, their hands or feet were blue, cold, and extremely painful. Perhaps no truer demonstration of the power of the emotions to cause physical pain exists than CRPS or migraine headaches. When patients and their parents come to accept and understand that relationship and agree to let a psychotherapist help them with those emotions, we are well on the road to healing—if not completely, at least to a better quality of life.

PSYCHOTHERAPY: A CRITICAL ELEMENT

As I've mentioned before, psychotherapy is a critical part of the treatment program for nearly every child in chronic pain, not just because psychological factors may be playing a role in the child's condition but also because the pain often has significant psychological effects on the child and the family. Anxiety, fear, uncertainty, resentment, depression, anger—all of these feelings and more can increase the sense of pain and make treatment efforts more difficult. If a child stubs a toe during an exciting soccer match, chances are he will brush off the incident and be back in the game in no time at all. But if a child has just been scolded by an angry parent or has lost his best friend and stubs his toe, now the same pain takes on huge proportions and will reduce the child to tears; the same injury, but not the same pain, and not the same suffering. What's the difference? The underlying emotional state.

Without professional psychological help, along with other treatments, patients cannot get the maximum benefit from their overall treatment program. In fact, individual and family counseling can be viewed as just another "dose" of medicine or biofeedback session. Psychiatry is about helping the child and family members unlock the body's natural powers to heal itself.

Having said that, I again want to emphasize that stress can increase or augment the child's experience of pain. That is, the pain itself is very real, and when you add the element of stress—be it fighting between parents, resentment from siblings, anxiety about trouble with schoolwork, feeling alienated from friends, poor self-esteem, worry about medical bills—pain worsens.

John's Story

Although the proper medications can provide significant pain relief for many youngsters, I also often have the privilege of witnessing the power of psychotherapy in helping improve the quality of life of a child who lives with chronic pain. Such is the case with John, who was brought to me by his parents, Arlene, a stay-at-home mom, and Josh, president of a software company, when he was ten years old. John has Charcot-Marie-Tooth disease, a degenerative neurologic disease characterized by muscle atrophy, especially in the legs, but also in the upper body, and significant neuropathic pain. The pain is associated with deterioration of the nerves and contractures that occur as part of the disease. In John's case, the pain makes it very difficult for him to participate in normal, everyday activities.

John had been to see several specialists, including neurologists, before he came to my office. When he came to me he was taking gabapentin (Neurontin) for the pain and Zoloft for anxiety disorder and depression. The gabapentin offered him little relief. In fact, he told me he had throbbing, aching pain in both feet and legs that usually ranked 8 out of 10, and that sometimes the pain was 10 out of 10.

Arlene told me that her son often cried out at night from the pain and that she would stay in bed with him until he fell asleep, which usually took two to three hours. Even then, the pain woke him up during the night, and so she usually stayed until dawn. In the meantime, John rarely got a good night's sleep, and he was exhausted during the day. He was attending school, and although he is extremely bright, he was doing poorly. I suspected a learning disorder, but since his school district had not given him the proper educational psychological testing as required by law, I had no accurate way at the time to make that determination.

After we conducted our intensive intake evaluation, I started John on a low dose of amitriptyline, which is not only effective in inducing and deepening sleep, but also helps relieve neuropathic pain. Then, because I try to avoid drug-drug interactions as much as possible, I immediately began to taper him off the gabapentin, which was not offering him any significant relief.

When John first came to see me, he had been seeing a psychotherapist for some time for his depression and anxiety disorder. While this therapy primarily involved dispensing and monitoring his medication, I thought one of the most important things we could do at that point was to initiate comprehensive psychotherapy with a child psychologist who had experience with pain management. John was going to have this disease for the rest of his life, and he needed to develop coping skills that he could rely on. At the same time, I was also concerned about Arlene's enmeshment with her son, including climbing into bed with him whenever he was in pain at night and allowing him to stay home from school more than seemed appropriate.

Although John's attachment and dependence on his mother was not great at age ten, it would become significant as time went on, and I was concerned that he would eventually be unable to become independent from her as he entered adolescence.

Both Arlene and Josh understood that some of their behaviors were holding John back from learning to cope with his pain on his own, and that he was getting a payback from that behavior; that is, he was getting extra attention, he was being allowed to stay home from school, and sometimes that also meant he would get special meals or privileges. They agreed to work with the child psychologist on their pain management behaviors, and John began to learn coping and distraction techniques. Six weeks later he returned to the clinic and reported that he was sleeping much better. Arlene and Josh were following the psychologist's suggestions and she had stopped running to John's room at night when he cried out. They were also more insistent about his going to school. However, John's pain had not improved significantly, and he continued to have a lot of anxiety, especially concerning school.

Rather than add another medication to work on his pain, I decided further psychological management was the best route. In addition to continuing his work with the child psychologist on coping and distracting skills, I arranged for John to see a neuropsychologist, who conducted comprehensive neuropsychiatric testing to define the nature of his learning disorder. If we could identify his learning difficulty, I told his parents, we could make adjustments to his schoolwork and thus reduce the stress associated with it. That, in turn, would improve his ability to manage his pain.

Over the next few months, I saw great improvements in

John and his family, especially the relationship between John and his mother. Her ability to recognize that some of her well-intended behaviors were actually hurting her son and her willingness to work with the child psychologist to modify them were instrumental in helping John develop the skills he would need for the rest of his life. John has incorporated deep breathing, progressive relaxation, and guided imagery into his life, and by using them both at home and in school he usually manages to keep his pain level less than 4 during the day. The neuropsychological testing uncovered some difficulties with comprehension, and John now receives special tutoring at school. With the improvements in his pain, sleep, and school work, John's anxiety and depression are well managed, and he and his family are anticipating a much brighter future.

THE "MISSED" DIAGNOSIS: WHAT PARENTS WORRY ABOUT

When eight-year-old Neela began to experience unexplained migrating pain—mostly joint pain, but occasional abdominal pain—her parents, Todd and Marsha, took her to their pediatrician who, after a thorough examination, could find no physical reason for the child's discomfort. The doctor prescribed acetaminophen and referred them to a child psychologist.

Neela's parents were not pleased. "The doctor just dismissed our daughter's pain and as much as told us it was all in her head," said Marsha. "It seemed as if he thought we were all crazy. But we know something must be wrong or else Neela wouldn't be having so much pain. What is the doctor missing?" Todd and Marsha became frustrated and fought with each other over what the doctor had said. They decided to seek a second opinion, and when the second doctor arrived at the same "nondiagnosis" and recommended antidepressants, they turned to the Internet and scoured it for yet another doctor. Again, they got the same news: the third doctor found nothing, suggested the symptoms were caused by stress, and referred them to a child psychologist.

Neela's Story

Todd and Marsha demonstrated a frequent concern of some parents of children in chronic pain: that the doctors have missed something. Although Todd and Marsha's deep concern for their child was obvious, they allowed their anxiety over thinking that the doctors had missed something to overshadow adequate treatment for their daughter. While her parents were doctor shopping, Neela was caught in the middle, receiving no real treatment and becoming more and more anxious as she watched her parents become increasingly upset with each other and with the doctors. The additional stress caused Neela to experience even more severe and frequent pain, which finally drove Todd and Marsha to follow the advice of the third doctor.

When the family met with a child psychologist, he immediately reassured them that he would be in regular contact with Neela's doctor and would keep a close eye on her symptoms. The psychologist began working with Neela on guided imagery and visualization, which helped her sleep much better, and he showed Marsha how to coach Neela through her sessions. After several months of seeing the psychologist, Neela developed bouts of bloody diarrhea, and she went back to her doctor for an abdominal sonogram and lower intestinal studies.

Based on the tests results and Neela's symptoms, the doctor diagnosed Crohn's disease, which sometimes has joint problems as an initial symptom. Immediately Todd and Marsha expressed their anger and asked how this condition could have been missed by the two previous doctors. Their current practitioner explained that many times, especially in children who have abdominal or joint pain, the condition is not apparent at first. Crohn's disease cannot be diagnosed by a blood test, only by taking a biopsy of the large intestine. Thus, until Neela experienced symptoms clearly related to her large intestine, bloody diarrhea, there was no logical rationale for taking a biopsy from there. Months, sometimes years pass before an accurate diagnosis can be made.

Parents need to understand that it is better to have an accurate diagnosis than a hasty one that may be incorrect. Not having a diagnosis, not knowing exactly what is wrong with your child, and wondering if the doctors have missed something can be a very frustrating and anxiety-producing time. During those uncertain times, however, it's important that the hurting child be treated on both a physical and mental/emotional level to relieve the symptoms until a more definitive picture of the situation can be found.

HOW TO RELATE TO A CHILD IN PAIN

When your child is in pain, your instinct as a parent or another close loved one is to protect and nurture him or her. You want to do everything in your power to make the pain go away and make your child happy and carefree. But you are dealing with chronic pain, and you don't want to make promises you can't keep. You can't promise your son that he'll never have another migraine or your daughter that when she wakes up in the morning, her CRPS will be gone forever. What you can do, however, is help your child develop critical emotional and social coping skills, such as self-esteem, inner strength, self-confidence, and poise.

Experts agree that children who live with chronic pain should be encouraged to view their condition as a challenge to be overcome rather than a burden or something that makes them "less than" other people. Thus it is important for your child to understand that you and other family members view her as an individual who is capable of managing and overcoming this challenge, as someone who is strong, not weak, someone who should be admired, not pitied. This doesn't mean you try to convince your child that she is better than everyone else. You need to emphasize your child's strengths and competence rather than focus on the illness.

Remember that your child is *not* the illness, and vice versa. Children with chronic pain should be encouraged and praised when they display health-promoting behaviors, such as practicing their coping skills. Rather than focus on pain as an excuse to miss school, for example, your child should be encouraged to attend and then rewarded with praise. Your words and actions let your child know you respect him and acknowledge that going to school and doing homework in the presence of pain is difficult, and that you respect and admire his efforts.

Naturally, this assumes that you are also pursuing treatment options that include coping skills to minimize or eliminate the pain. You should consider this "tough love" approach to be part of your child's treatment program as well. If your child must live with chronic pain for a period of time, whether it be weeks, months, or even years, you have an obligation to make her life as normal as possible. "Normal" means your child should go to school whenever possible, maintain contact with friends, participate in school, social, and family activities as much as possible, and be encouraged to practice coping skills rather than succumb to pain and disability behaviors (e.g., not wanting to go to school, staying away from friends, allowing the pain to control her life). If you are an adult with pain, your goal is to get back to work. For the child with pain, her work is to learn and develop, and to do this she must go to school and function in the social environment of her peers.

Bobbie's Story

Bobbie is an eight-year-old boy who lives with his mother, stepfather, and two older stepbrothers. He had been experiencing chronic headaches for more than six months before his mother, Katelynn, brought him to my pain management center. Before coming here, she had taken him to his pediatrician, who had referred her to a neurologist. The neurologist found nothing physically wrong, prescribed ibuprofen, and recommended a child psychologist. Katelynn accepted the prescriptions but declined the suggestion of a psychologist.

During the first six months of Bobbie's headache complaints, Katelynn used to let him stay home from school every time he complained. When the complaints came every day, even though Bobbie was on medication, she didn't know what to do, and contemplated home schooling. As it became obvious that Bobbie would not graduate into the next grade and his headaches were causing more and more friction in the household, Katelynn decided to get a second opinion. That's when she and Bobbie came to see me.

My examination also revealed nothing physically wrong with Bobbie, but it was clear he was a nervous child. Whenever I asked him a question, he would always look at his mother and wait for her to answer, and he always stayed next to his mother. I asked them both to keep a pain diary, and then I strongly recommended he and his mother see a child psychologist as part of our overall therapeutic package, and Katelynn agreed.

After Katelynn and Bobbie had a few sessions with the psychologist, Katelynn began to understand how allowing Bobbie to stay home from school whenever he complained of a headache was doing him more harm than good. Katelynn also came to realize that Bobbie's headaches had started right after she had remarried and Bobbie had acquired two new older stepbrothers. Bobbie's headaches and insistence on staying home from school seemed to be his way of maintaining his close and exclusive relationship with his mother, which he had enjoyed for six of his eight years after Katelynn's divorce.

The psychologist met alone with Katelynn and Bobbie's stepfather, Ken, and gave them tips on how they could begin to help Bobbie become more independent and confident, and more in control of his pain instead of allowing the pain to rule his life. Part of what Katelynn and Ken needed to do was to encourage Bobbie to practice his coping skills, which the psychologist had been on working with Bobbie, showing him how to do breathing exercises and progressive relaxation. The psychologist also instructed them to try to keep Bobbie on as regular a routine as possible, and to also balance the time each of them spent with all three of their children.

Katelynn tried her new strategy the next time Bobbie wanted to stay home from school. Although she said it was difficult at first, "because I felt I was being mean," she was firm. "Bobbie, I know you're not feeling well, but I know you can do your relaxation exercises to help you with the pain. Why don't you practice them right now, and then come downstairs for breakfast and get ready for school."

When Bobbie returns from school each day, Katelynn sits down with him and asks him about his day. If he has a headache, she suggests he practice his relaxation exercises. Then, as she and the psychologist had discussed, she places a sticker on the calendar on Bobbie's wall in his room to show that he attended school that day. Every time he completes an entire week of school, he can choose from a special list of treats he and Katelynn had agreed upon, such as getting to choose the video the family will watch on Friday night, or being allowed to stay up until ten on weekends. Katelynn has also reinstituted Bobbie's chores, which before the headaches began had included taking out the trash and making his bed every day. Both Katelynn and her husband make sure Bobbie keeps up his chores, and do offer to help him—but not do them for him—if he's not feeling well.

After more than two months, Katelynn says that Bobbie has improved a lot. "His headaches are significantly better, and he's so proud when he completes an entire week of school. I keep telling him that in no time, he'll have his headaches beat, that he's strong enough to do it, and I think he's beginning to believe it too." Ken has been doing his part as well by taking all three boys to baseball and soccer games when Bobbie is feeling well.

SUPPORT GROUPS

We talked about the importance of support groups in Chapter 3, but here I want to mention them again because they can be instrumental in helping family members understand and cope with a child who has chronic pain. Whether you attend a live group session or visit chat rooms online, the emotional support you can get from sharing your experiences and concerns, or just listening to others, can be invaluable.

"I didn't know anyone else who had a child with juvenile rheumatoid arthritis," said Bernadette. "I'm a single mom, I work full time, and I spend every spare moment with my son, Ricky, who is eight. The stress of caring for Ricky was getting to me, and none of my friends understood, although they meant well. Being able to go online at night and chat and correspond with other mothers who have JRA kids is a lifesaver. I've become great friends with several of these women, and we all support each other. A few of us are even going to get together with our kids some day soon. I know I'm a better mom for Ricky because of their support."

Going to support groups or talks given by relevant organizations, such as the Arthritis Foundation or the Endometriosis Association, or participating in online chats can benefit all members of the family. Siblings, grandparents, aunts and uncles, cousins—anyone who is intimately involved in the child's life or who wants to better understand the situation can find answers from these groups and organizations. (See the Appendix for a list of support group contacts.)

BOTTOM LINE

One of the best therapies for a child who has chronic pain is to be surrounded by loving, supportive people in a peaceful environment. This is a prescription that you can't put into a capsule or injection. To provide such an environment, parents of a hurting child need to look at how the chronic pain situation is affecting the family dynamics and then strive to restore them to as normal a state as possible.

If you cut your finger, your body reacts by discharging platelets to the wound site to try to stop the blood flow. Calcium, blood proteins, and fibrinogen then help the platelets to form a clot. The clot then interacts with blood cells to form a scab. Eventually the scab falls off and the skin is healed and returns to normal. When you have a child with chronic or persistent pain, you are frantic to help. All of your emotions are focused on this desire to help. You stay on alert all the time, your stress level is high, and you may neglect other areas of your life (including your spouse, other children, job, school, friends). A scab of resentment, anger, fear, depression, hopelessness, and anxiety appears and keep growing. Unless you do something about it, the scab won't fall off and allow healing to occur.

To help keep your entire family healthy, you need to manage the stress and anxiety that often build around a child who is in pain. As we've discussed, some ways to do that are:

- Maintain as normal a family life as possible. Evaluate your current family situation, compare it with how life was before chronic pain became a part of your child's life, and take steps to bring the family back into balance. This may mean you need to make a list of how specific situations were before and how they are now, and then you can focus on a plan.
- Seek support. Psychotherapy is a critical part of the healing process for both the children and their parents. Support groups can also lend emotional help.
- Encourage coping behaviors rather than pain behaviors. Children who regularly practice coping skills, such as biofeedback, progressive relaxation, self-hypnosis, guided imagery, and meditation, experience less stress, and as a result, so do other family members.
- Promote positive thinking. Although your hurting child may feel he or she is different or weird, it is important that all family members emphasize that the pain is a challenge that can be managed, and that the hurting child has their support in accepting that challenge.
- Balance the time you spend with all your children. Siblings may feel resentful, shut out, angry, or frightened if you appear to favor the hurting child. Based on their level of understanding, siblings should be told about the chronic pain condition and be allowed to share their feelings about it and their brother or sister with you in a nonthreatening environment. If you feel uneasy about such conversations, you may want to talk to a psychologist, who can help you initiate such talks with your children.

Chapter 8

HELPING YOUR CHILD THRIVE OUTSIDE THE HOME

Part of the quest to restore childhood to children who live with chronic pain includes giving them the tools they need to *be* children. Childhood involves many activities—going to school, playing with friends, learning how to share, enjoying vacations, playing sports, making new discoveries about the world. For some children, chronic or recurring pain can mar each of these joys of childhood. But you can change that.

Your role, with the help of the medical professionals who work with you, is to teach your child how to live as comfortably, successfully, and joyfully as possible while learning how to care for him or herself. This means you will need to recognize what your child's physical and emotional limits are and, depending on the age of your child, allow him or her to recognize them as well. A five-year-old child with juvenile rheumatoid arthritis may play too long and hard and end up in bed for a week unless you monitor his or her activity, yet a teenager should be allowed to decide what toll staying up late with friends or going to the mall will have on his or her pain and energy levels and take responsibility for decisions that affect them. That's not to say that the five-year-old should not be taught responsibility, but the amount of understanding and responsibility you can expect from a younger child will be less than that of an older one.

In this chapter you can learn how to help your child function and thrive in the world. We will discuss how to talk to your child about chronic pain and the condition that is causing it. We will explore ways to equip your child with self-confidence and coping skills he or she will need to engage in normal childhood activities such as sports, play dates with friends, school field trips, parties, and social gatherings, including how to choose activities that are most appropriate for them, how to know when to say *no,* how to ask for help from other adults, how to recognize and accept any limitations and challenges they may encounter, and how to feel comfortable with themselves—and have fun—in social situations. Lastly, we will explain how to foster good communication with and enlist the support and help of teachers, school administrators, and adults in charge of your child's school and recreation.

WHY DO I HURT? TALKING TO YOUR CHILD ABOUT PAIN

Seven-year-old Tommy sat at the desk, carefully coloring in a picture of himself and his family he had just drawn. The child psychologist sat next to him and pointed to the jagged black and green lines coming out of the head of the picture Tommy had made of himself. "What are those lines, Tommy?" The child cocked his head and mumbled, "my headache."

"So is the pain leaving your head and going away into space?" Tommy shook his head. The psychologist tried again. "What are the lines doing?" Tommy picked up a crayon and started to draw more green lines around his head. "They're hitting my head and making it hurt."

"Why do you think they're doing that?" the psychologist asked. Tommy shrugged and kept on drawing. "I guess I did something bad."

Pain As Punishment

Younger children are more likely to think they are having pain because they've done something wrong, while older children usually understand that they are not responsible for their pain. Both groups of children will experience frustration, however, and how they express it can differ depending on several factors, including the child's age, intelligence level, family situation, ability to manage the pain, and degree of support from family and other sources.

According to Julie Collier, PhD, in private practice in Palo Alto, California, and formerly the pediatric pain psychologist with the Lucile Packard Children's Hospital, explaining to a child why he or she has chronic pain is usually not a major sticking point for most children and their families. Although some children, like Tommy, may believe they have done something wrong to deserve the pain they feel, this misconception can be erased by parents, with the help of a mental health professional if need be, by gently and repeatedly over time reassuring the child that he or she has done nothing to cause the pain and that the pain is caused by something else. Then, depending on the child's level of understanding, the parent can explain, say, what a migraine is, what happens in the body to cause the pain, and that many people, children and adults, get migraines and that none of them has done anything wrong.

Tommy's psychologist spoke with Tracy, Tommy's mother, and learned that Tommy's migraine attacks had started around the time she and her husband had gotten a divorce. When the psychologist questioned Tommy further, he told her that "Daddy yelled at Mommy and he yelled at me and then I yelled at him and then he left. I made Daddy leave."

The psychologist then instructed Tommy's mother to use a two-step approach to help change Tommy's ideas about the cause of his pain. Once a day, Tracy was to tell Tommy that "you didn't make Daddy leave. Mommy and Daddy decided to live in different places and we both love you very much." She was to incorporate this message into their daily routine, without drawing too much attention to it, but yet making sure her son understood. Tracy found that the best time to deliver the reinforcement was at bedtime, when she was giving her son a good night hug and kiss.

Tracy was also instructed to explain to Tommy how migraines worked. Tracy asked one of the nurses in the doctor's office to help her with the migraine explanation, and they found some pictures of the brain and blood vessels that Tommy could color. Within a few weeks, Tommy was drawing pictures of a brain and bulging blood vessels and telling the psychologist "that's why I hurt."

Denying the Pain

For some children, especially adolescents, accepting their chronic pain condition is extremely difficult, and they try to deny that it is part of their life. Sixteen-year-old Natalie, who was first diagnosed with fibromyalgia when she was twelve, admits she fights with her mother about accepting her condition. "My mother is always on me about taking my medication, and I really hate to take it," she says. "Even when I'm in a lot of pain and I know the painkillers will relieve it, I still argue with my mom about it. I know she's right, that the medicine will help, but it's just not fair. Why does this disease control me? Why can't I control it? At least when I refuse to take my meds, even if it's only for a few hours, that's when I'm in control. I know it's stupid, but that's how I feel."

Natalie's frustration and anger are not unusual, especially among teenagers. They are mature and intelligent enough to understand the medical explanation of why they have chronic pain, but that doesn't mean they like it and won't fight and deny it all they can. In some ways this rebellion is healthy; children like Natalie are determined to live a better life, to be normal like their friends. While they are rebelling against and denying their condition, they are also learning their limitations (see "Recognizing Limitations" below).

The Truth Hurts Less

Whether children with chronic pain are in kindergarten or high school, they deserve to know why they have pain. Naturally, the explanation needs to be at a level they can understand. Tommy's mother Tracy understood this, earlier in this chapter, when she explained why he had migraine pain, and it's what you can do as well. Like Tracy, you may want to ask your doctor, nurse, or other health professional who is familiar with your child's condition how to explain it. One approach, which works well with young children, is to ask them to draw their pain, and then use the drawing to explain what is really happening. In that way, your child can learn to see his or her own creation in a new light. Or, you can explain the pain to your child and then ask him or her to draw it for you. This approach also gives your child ownership of the pain, and the drawing can be a starting point for guided imagery or biofeedback sessions.

Older children can usually understand a more sophisticated explanation. Your doctor or therapist may have some materials that can help you with the explanation, including reading material or models. You may also want to get literature, videos, books, and other information from organizations that focus on the condition that affects your child; for example, the American Council for Headache Education, or the Endometriosis Association, or the Arthritis Foundation. Some organizations have support groups and offer talks that may help both you and your child better understand the cause of the chronic pain.

When Pain Doesn't Get Better

Another thing about pain that is difficult for children—and adults—to understand is why, after trying several different drugs, sometimes the pain doesn't get any better. This can create a lot of stress, anxiety, and anger: children can get angry at their parents and their doctors, parents may blame the doctors and each other, and there can be increased tension between children and their parents. Both children and their parents may begin to feel helpless and hopeless. If children need to undergo uncomfortable tests or therapy, this can add to the negative feelings.

Children with chronic pain also need to cope with knowing that the condition they have may, depending on what it is, be permanent and may even get worse. Child and adolescent psychiatrists note that many of these children initially refuse to believe they are ill, and then become angry later on. Emotional support for both children and parents from psychologists or other mental health professionals, as well as support groups and organizations, is critical for helping children and their families get through these difficult feelings.

When Kids Tell Other Kids about Their Pain

"What's wrong with you? Why can't you go skateboarding any more?" "Why are you always sick?" "Why did you quit the team?" The time will come—if it hasn't already—when your child will be asked questions like these by his or her classmates or friends. The remarks may even be hurtful, such as "What's wrong, are you a wuss?" or "You're just a big baby," or "You don't have the guts to go out for the team." And your first instinct may be to jump in and explain why your child can't play football today or go on an overnight camping trip or skateboard in the park.

It's important that you respect your child's wishes when it comes to how, when, and what other children know about your child's health. Children who are comfortable or who have come to terms with their limitations are more likely to discuss their health problems with their friends, even if only one or two of their closest ones. However, they must do so in their own time and on their own terms. You can offer to help them by asking them to share with you how they feel about their health and about their friends knowing about it. At the same time, you should emphasize that you will not betray their confidence and tell their friends if they do not want you to.

If you have a young child with chronic pain that limits her

activities, you might talk to your child's friends' parents about your child's limitations. Using this approach, the parents can talk to their children, and your child is spared having to explain why she can't go bike riding with the rest of the kids or why he can't play more than a few innings of baseball. If your child's teachers need to know about the health problems, you should make sure they know they are not to discuss the nature of your child's condition with anyone.

Allowing your child to talk about his condition with friends and classmates may seem like a small thing. But for a child who has pain that is difficult to control, having the option to control who, when, and what he tells others about it is no small deal. Children face the risk of losing friends when they reveal—and admit—that they are different than their peers. If this happens, you will need to empathize with his loss and to focus on those friends who are accepting of his limitations. This may also be a good time to suggest going to a support group or to find ways for your child to share time with other children who have similar health problems, such as camp for children with arthritis or a social event sponsored by a support group or an organization that deals with your child's condition. See the Appendix for a list of organizations and support groups.

EQUIPPING YOUR CHILD TO THRIVE IN THE WORLD

Children who live with chronic pain have an extra layer of coping to deal with in their lives. Besides absorbing all there is to learn about their environment at home, in school, and the rest of the world, they have this thing called "pain" that keeps tugging at their sleeve, trying to bring them down. As parents you can do much to equip your hurting children with ways to shrug away the pain and to cope, even thrive, in their world. While building physical strength, flexibility, and endurance are important, strengthening the mind and fortifying the spirit are equally if not more critical for these children. Here are some steps you can take to help your children meet the mental and spiritual challenges they face.

Listen to Your Child's Concerns

Children have a right to have their feelings validated by others, especially by their parents and their caregivers. Although such validation doesn't make the pain go away, there is comfort in knowing that others believe and understand you. This is true for adults as well as children. Because pain is, in the final analysis, a private and subjective experience, if children say they have pain, we must believe them. We must never deny the existence of pain that children tell us they have. If we want them to continue with their activities, go to school, and so on, then we must acknowledge their pain and their feelings while stating how they will continue with their activities.

Once children are old enough to express their thoughts, they can tell you what is bothering them. A four-year-old and a fourteen-year-old will articulate their fears, anger, and other emotions at different levels of sophistication, yet it's important that you allow your child the opportunity to express her feelings about her friends, school, playing sports, being around strangers, going on school trips, and other activities away from home. Children should be allowed to talk about these concerns in a relaxed, open setting, in which they can speak freely, without anyone passing judgment or interrupting. Some children, especially younger ones, may need some encouragement to speak or some leading questions to help them express themselves. The questions should either give children some options or help them verbalize the thoughts in their head.

For example, eight-year-old Justin has frequent flare-ups of juvenile rheumatoid arthritis that are never severe enough to keep him out of school. But after his most recent episode soon after the beginning of the new school year, he insisted he didn't want to go to school. At first his mother, Linda, was concerned that he was in too much pain to get around in school, but she noticed that he was moving around the house in a way that was similar to when he had had previous flare-ups.

Linda's next thought was to reassure Justin that he would be okay in school and to insist that he go. But she also knew that not wanting to go to school was uncharacteristic of her son, so she made him his favorite dessert and while they sat and ate it, she asked him questions about school, trying to sound as nonchalant as possible.

After about fifteen minutes, Justin revealed that some of his classmates were teasing him about limping, and that he was having trouble getting to his classes in the crowded hallways. Sometimes he also got so stiff while sitting in class that he had a very hard time getting out of his chair. Justin said he felt "weird" and different and didn't want to go to school anymore.

Linda found it difficult to sit and listen to her son tell her how he felt, because she wanted to interrupt and say "Why didn't you tell me this sooner?" But she let him talk and only interjected a few comments, like "What do the other children say to you?" and "It sounds like school has been hard for you this year," and "We need to find ways to help you feel better about going to school," and "Tell me about anything else that bothers you at school."

Like Linda, you need to open the door of communication between yourself and your child and, at least at first, let the communication be mostly one-way. Choose a comfortable and nonthreatening setting where you won't be interrupted. One mom chose to talk to her twelve-year-old daughter about her fibromyalgia while they were driving to the mall to buy clothes. Nine-year-old Nelson was on a fishing trip with his dad when they talked about his migraines. Fifteen-year-old Becky talked about her endometriosis when her mom took her out for ice cream one night.

Involve Your Child in the Solution

Once you know how your child feels and the types of challenges he or she is facing, it's time to find solutions. Children should be involved in this process, as they are much more likely to benefit if they agree to the solutions. Even young children can have a say.

First, you should be clear about what the problem is. In Justin's case, there were challenges at school that made him want to stay home. Solutions, therefore, would involve removing or reducing those challenges so going to school would be more pleasant.

Once you can define the problem, ask your child what she thinks some solutions are. Young children like Justin probably won't have an answer, but it's important that children feel they are involved in the process. When Justin said "I don't know how to fix it," Linda made some suggestions. "What if we find a way for you to leave class a little bit early so you can get to your next class on time?" Justin liked that idea. Linda also suggested that Justin might be allowed to get up several times during class so he wouldn't get stiff from sitting too long. Because these suggestions required cooperation from Justin's teachers, Linda made an appointment to speak with each of them, and they all agreed to let Justin leave class a few minutes early and to let him get up during class—to help pass out papers, get a drink of water, get supplies from the closet—to help keep him limber.

Linda hoped that the teasing from other students would improve once Justin was able to get around school better. Justin's doctor suggested he might talk with a child psychologist and that Justin might benefit from being around other children who have juvenile rheumatoid arthritis. Linda contacted her local branch of the Arthritis Foundation and learned about a support group and a camp for children with JRA.

Getting your child involved with a support group or other children who share his or her condition can help with self-esteem. When children see there are other children like themselves, they feel less alone, less different, and better about themselves. (See "Support Groups" in Chapter 3.) They talk about their experiences and how they have learned to cope with pain and being different than their friends.

Adolescents can be especially resistant to suggestions from parents and health-care practitioners about how to find solutions to their challenges. Fourteen-year-old Christy had been very reluctant to discuss with her mother the pelvic pain she was experiencing. Once she did admit to her mother that she felt "totally weird" around her friends, she said she didn't want to talk about it anymore.

"My heart went out to her, and I wanted so much to help her," said her mother, Sarah. "But she wouldn't open up. I suggested we go shopping together so we could talk, and she refused to talk. So every day I said to her, 'I'd love to help you find some ways to deal with your feelings about this, so if you can think of some things that might work, we can talk about it.' I don't know if she just got tired of hearing me say it every day, but after about a week, she blurted out 'I just feel so alone, like no one believes me, like I'm weird, like this will never go away.' And that was the beginning of our dialogue."

At that point, Sarah gave Christy information on how to contact support groups and online chats where she could communicate with many girls who were going through experiences similar to hers. "I left it up to Christy to make the next move," said Sarah. "I knew I couldn't do it for her. I could hear her on her computer in her room late at night, and after a few days she told me about this 'cool site' for teenagers who have endometriosis and how she can correspond with other girls just like her. Now her whole attitude has changed. She's even told a few of her friends about the endometriosis sites, and now they understand what she goes through. It was important for Christy to do this on her terms; all I had to do was give her some tools to work with."

Encourage Coping Skills

Your child can better thrive in the world and get through difficult challenges once he learns and practices coping skills. We have talked about many such skills in this book, including biofeedback, meditation, guided imagery, relaxation, distraction, and self-hypnosis. You've seen how critical they can be in helping children who have chronic pain, and the truth is that not only are these skills helpful today, but for many children, they will be needed for many years to come, perhaps their entire lives.

But these skills are only useful if your child uses them. That may mean you will need to gently remind your daughter or son to turn to these practices when they are in pain. Again we return to Justin, who was taught self-hypnosis and progressive relaxation by his psychologist. When Justin becomes upset about being unable to play with his friends or about having to go to school, he often forgets to use these skills, because the most important thing to him at that moment is how he feels emotionally. Fortunately, his mother understands how the stress Justin feels contributes to his pain, and so she immediately reminds him to practice his coping skills.

RECOGNIZING LIMITATIONS

Every child can expect to have days when he or she doesn't feel well enough to play with friends or go to the mall or ride a bike. But for children who have chronic pain, there may be many of those days. You need to make every effort to see that your child continues to live as normal a lifestyle as possible.

As we discussed, it's important that children be involved in making decisions about how to work out their challenges.

Helping children to recognize their limitations and then allowing them to take responsibility for their decisions can be one of the hardest things parents do. In the long run, however, it teaches them to balance their lives, to take responsibility for their decisions, and to feel self-confident and independent.

Gary's Story

Cora admits her twelve-year-old son, Gary, is a handful. Diagnosed with sickle cell anemia when he was less than a year old, he has always been what his mother calls "a fighter." "He has one younger and one older brother, and he tries to keep up with them all the time. When he was younger, I really limited his activities. I was so afraid he would get too tired or overheated or dehydrated. As he got older, he didn't want to listen to me anymore. The harder I tried to set limits, the more he resented it. He got angry once and told me to stop treating him like he was sick. I knew he wanted to be one of the crowd, to play basketball and ride his bike and be with his friends. But I also was afraid what it would do to him."

Cora talked to her doctor, and he said she should treat her son as normally as possible, to encourage him to monitor his own activities and to let Gary know that she would support his decisions, but that he would reap the consequences of them.

"Gary has had eight sickle cell crises, so he knows how bad the pain can be," said Cora. "And I know that deep down he knows his own limitations. Once I started to allow him to limit himself, even though it was very hard for me to do, I saw a difference. When he's tired, he'll come home right after school instead of playing ball at the park. I've heard him turn down invitations to go to the mall with his friends. He's listening to his body, and that's good. I never say anything about the times he decides to stay home. And I also keep my mouth shut when he does too much and he pays for it the next few days. But he knows I'm there to support him, no matter what, and our relationship is better for it. I'd rather have my son remember his adolescence in a positive way, even though he may not feel well sometimes, than to grow up resenting me and not learning how to set his own limitations."

Megan's Story

Younger children usually need a bit more guidance in setting limitations. Seven-year-old Megan, for example, used to get very upset when she couldn't play in the treehouse or ride bikes with her friends when her juvenile rheumatoid arthritis flared. Her well-intentioned parents, Bob and Pat, would keep her in the house and try to comfort her with promises of videos and her favorite foods, but Megan would cry for hours and end up exhausted, while her parents' nerves were frayed.

When Bob and Pat mentioned these emotional episodes to the child psychologist, he pointed out that they would likely have much better success if they found ways to make their daughter feel less "different" by choosing activities she could do with her friends. For example, since Megan couldn't climb into the treehouse, where her friends would have tea parties with their dolls, she could invite the girls over for a tea party in the house. Bob and Pat then put up a tent in their basement, and the girls felt like they were in a special place just for them. The psychologist also noted that Megan's physical therapist had recommended swimming, and said that enrolling Megan in a swimming program with other children would be not only therapeutic but fun as well.

He also suggested that Bob and Pat talk to Megan about making a list of activities she could do when her condition flared, things she could do either alone or when she invited friends over. Together they created a list: making puzzles, drawing, painting with water colors, cutting out pictures and making a collage, and stringing beads.

Managing the Condition

In Chapter 1, I mentioned that although parents' response to a child who has chronic or recurring pain is usually done with the best of intentions, the response often is also inappropriate or even detrimental. And this is understandable. Think about your own situation. Do you find that, because you care so much about your child, you may panic or become excessively worried about your child's condition and, as a result, you are overprotective?

Take Bryanne, for example. Bryanne is a bright thirteen-year-old girl who was diagnosed with fibromyalgia around her twelfth birthday. Prior to the diagnosis, she and her mother, Sandra, had been to numerous doctors over nearly a two-year period, searching for the reason behind the chronic fatigue, periodic dizziness, sleep problems, and pain that plagued the young girl. During the years of doctor hopping, Sandra had grown increasingly concerned and protective, and the result was that she catered to Bryanne's every whim.

For example, if Bryanne said she was too tired to go to

school, Sandra let her stay home, where she played video games, watched television, and slept. "I don't want her to overexert herself at school," said Sandra. Sandra would try to "cheer up" her daughter by bringing home pizzas and ice cream, two of her daughter's favorite foods. Although several doctors had suggested that Bryanne would feel better if she got some regular exercise (even though they hadn't offered a diagnosis), Bryanne always insisted she was too tired to take a walk or play with the dog, and Sandra let her daughter have her way.

By the time Bryanne got her diagnosis, she was overweight, deconditioned, and depressed. The doctor was very encouraging, telling Sandra and Bryanne that fibromyalgia, although challenging, could be managed with guidelines she could easily incorporate into her daily life. He emphasized that children who have fibromyalgia can still grow up relatively normally and engage in many of the activities their friends participate in, though in modified forms at times.

One of the first things the doctor recommended was counseling for both Bryanne and her mother, separately and together. The psychologist helped them both deal with the feelings of anger and frustration they had about the fibromyalgia and the limitations it was putting on Bryanne. Bryanne learned that she could channel those feelings into constructive activities, such as learning to play the flute for the school orchestra or drawing. Sandra also learned something. "At first I didn't want to hear it or believe it, but the psychologist showed me how I was channeling all my concern for Bryanne into things that actually were hurting her, like letting her skip school whenever she said she was too tired to go, or not walk the dog and get some exercise. I thought I was showing her how much I cared, but my actions were actually detrimental, such as giving in to Bryanne whenever she didn't want to exercise or go to school."

The doctor also assigned a physical therapist to work with Bryanne and start her on an exercise program that would build muscle tone and strength without tiring her out. Since Bryanne had some friends who played on the school volleyball team, Sandra and the therapist spoke with the volleyball coach and worked out a schedule where she could practice with the other girls at least part of each session and act as scorekeeper the rest of the time. This allowed Bryanne to get some exercise and have fun at the same time, and also socialize with her friends. Once she started getting more active, she lost some weight, began to feel better about herself, and was less depressed.

On days Bryanne is too fatigued for a whole day of school, Sandra has prearranged with the school for her daughter to attend at least half a day, and for her to bring the rest of her work home.

GOING TO SCHOOL

The job of childhood is to acquire knowledge and experiences while developing social skills. Therefore, attending school is critically important for all children, not only to get an education, but to develop the self-confidence and the social skills they will need to succeed as adults. If your child is having difficulty while attending school or is missing a lot of days because of chronic pain, there are steps you can take to help your child do the very best he or she can in school. This often means you need to talk or meet with your child's teachers and other school personnel so everyone understands what your child's limitations may be and what can be done to meet them.

The Right to an Education

Every child in the United States, regardless of his or her special needs, has a right to receive free and equal public education. These rights are granted per the Individuals with Disabilities Education Act of 1990. It's up to you to contact your child's educators so you can work together to allow your child to participate in classroom and other school activities as much as possible, and it's up to the school to devise a plan that will accommodate the needs of your child. Sometimes that means some adjustments will need to be made in terms of transportation to and from school, time needed to get from class to class, time off for medical appointments, medications that need to be taken during the day, or time out during the day for therapy. These and other modifications can be worked out once you understand what your child's needs are in the school environment.

Other times, a plan for your child may mean something more. It is not unusual for children with chronic pain to miss months or even years of school. During this extended period of school absence, most school systems will develop a home school program, but the effectiveness of home schooling will depend upon the ability of your child to learn, and the level of commitment of the teachers and school leaders. As mentioned in Chapter 3, child psychologists can perform formal educational testing, which will inform both you and the school district of your child's level of performance. This information will then allow the psychologist, school officials, and you to develop a custom educational program that will allow your child to maintain his or her school work on par with the rest of the class, or a program to allow your child to catch up to the level at which he or she should be performing.

This kind of program is called an individual educational plan, or IEP. Most school districts are mandated by law to develop IEPs for children with handicaps or illnesses that prevent them from learning in a conventional fashion, but there is great variability in the quality and effectiveness of IEPs, depending upon whether the district follows through with their requirement, which is your child's legal right. If your child is missing a lot of school, is having difficulty keeping up with classwork because of his or her illness, or you have other concerns about your child's schoolwork, talk to your psychologist about the possible need for an IEP.

Identifying Your Child's Needs

Nine-year-old Louis gets migraines, fourteen-year-old Rheanne has CRPS, ten-year-old Richie has juvenile rheumatoid arthritis, and seven-year-old Sandra has spondylitis. Each one of these children has some special needs when it comes to their education, ranging from getting ready for school in the morning to moving from class to class, participating in recess or physical education, standing in line, concentrating in class, or opening a locker. You need to know what challenges your child faces before, during, and after school so you, your child, and school personnel can work together to minimize or eliminate them.

You can begin by asking your child what difficulties he or she has at school, but you will likely need to help identify those problems by asking some questions, especially if your child is in elementary school. Older children may be reluctant to talk about their problems at all, and so you may need to play detective to uncover them. To help you with that task, we have provided a list of questions you can use for children of any age and with any chronic pain condition (see box).

Whether your child is young or older, it is helpful to visit the school so you can observe the layout of the classrooms and other school areas and any obstacles that may affect your child. If possible, try to do this when other parents are on campus or when your child is not at school; most children are embarrassed to have mom and dad checking up on them in front of their peers. Make an appointment to speak with your child's teachers, either on the phone or in person, to discuss any difficulties they may have observed as well.

Working with School Personnel

Once you have identified your child's needs in the school environment, you can address them by enlisting the assistance of school personnel or, depending on what your child's challenges are, getting the cooperation of your child's health-care practitioner. For example, eleven-year-old Julia has juvenile rheumatoid arthritis, and she has trouble carrying her books and maneuvering down the crowded hallways. After her mother spoke with the principal and Julia's teachers and the doctor talked to the school nurse, Julia is now allowed to leave her classes a few minutes early so she can get to her next class without being jostled in a crowd, and there are several children who take turns carrying her books to class for her.

IDENTIFYING CHALLENGES IN YOUR CHILD'S SCHOOL ENVIRONMENT

This is a list of general questions; therefore, not all of them will apply to your child's situation. You can ask your child to answer the questions as well as make observations to answer them for yourself and also question your child's teachers. This list may also prompt you to think of others we have not included.

- Is it difficult for you to get to school?
- Do you have a problem getting on or riding on the bus?
- Do you have difficulty sitting for long periods of time?
- Do the overhead lights in the building bother you?
- Do you have sufficient time to get from class to class?
- Are the hallways too crowded for you to maneuver through easily and safely?
- Do you have a problem opening your locker?
- Do you have difficulty carrying your books and other supplies?
- Do you have trouble carrying a tray in the cafeteria?
- Are there any steps or stairways that are difficult for you to use?
- Are the bathrooms difficult for you to use?
- Do you get very tired any time during the day?
- Are you allowed to go to the nurse's office when you need to?
- Do you have trouble standing in line; for example, in the cafeteria?
- Are the chairs and desks comfortable for you?
- Does it bother you to have to take medicine during school hours?
- Do some of the other students make fun of you?
- Do some of the teachers treat you differently because you have health challenges?
- Do you have trouble writing and taking notes?
- Do you have difficulty changing clothes for PE class?

In some cases, such as when your child needs medication, your health-care practitioner should take part in helping develop a plan to help your child function better at school. Ten-year-old Jorge has chronic daily headache and occasional migraines. His doctor provided the school with Jorge's headache management plan, which included a list of the medications he was taking and the limits on how often he could take them, use of progressive relaxation exercises for twenty to thirty minutes when needed for pain control, and a request he be allowed to wear dark glasses in class because he is sensitive to the overhead lights. The school agreed to keep Jorge's parents informed of his medication use and to tell them immediately if Jorge displayed any unusual behaviors or need for medication.

Because the medication policy of each school is different, it is important that parents and their health-care practitioners discuss the school's regulations as early in the school year as possible so a workable plan can be put into place and the child can continue with classes and get any required medication with as little disruption as possible.

It may also be necessary for your health-care provider to inform school personnel about how much activity your child should participate in during recesses and physical education programs. If there are any special adaptations needed for writing, sitting, or moving about the halls or stairways, these should be discussed as well.

Whenever possible, it is best for children who have chronic pain to stay in school, learn to function in the presence of pain, and keep as normal an activity schedule as possible. Children who continue to go to school despite their pain learn to overcome personal obstacles, continue socialization, earn the respect of others and themselves, and learn to overcome fears related to their condition. Naturally, there are circumstances in which some children must be home schooled because of their chronic pain conditions, but in those cases it is critical that parents incorporate social activities with other children for their child so he will not feel isolated from his peers and become depressed.

Helping Your Child Communicate His or Her Needs

Some children need to take a short break or do relaxation exercises during the school day in order for them to stay in school all day. If your child has such needs, you will need to communicate this to all of her teachers, the principle, and the nurse. Your health-care practitioner may also alert the school nurse of these needs. School personnel should also tell you if any of them feel your child seems to be asking for more time off than necessary. Once school personnel are aware of and agree to the request, you need to make sure your child understands that she should communicate these requests to school officials in a clear and polite manner and only when necessary.

Marissa, for example, is a seventh-grader who has fibromyalgia. She hates to miss school, but some days she is so fatigued by midmorning, she can't stay awake. Her teachers know that she may ask for a brief break, and so she'll say, "I'm really tired, may I take a short break?" She spends about thirty minutes in the nurse's office and then returns to class. Some days she needs a break in the afternoon, while other days she is able to attend all her classes without leaving class.

COMMUNICATING WITH YOUR CHILD'S SCHOOL PERSONNEL

Here are a few guidelines on how to keep communication open between yourself and your child's teachers, principal, and other school personnel.

- Make an appointment to meet with your child's teacher(s) at least twice a year. These visits are in addition to any regular open house events, parent-teacher conferences, and chance meetings at school events. Send a note or email to the teacher(s) (not with your child!) to arrange such meetings.
- Ask how teachers and school personnel will keep you informed about your child's progress. Are there progress reports issued during the semester? When report cards are given out? On a weekly or monthly basis?
- If possible, volunteer at your child's school or participate in activities, such as helping at sporting events and bake sales, or being a teacher's aide.
- If you know your child is having trouble or you suspect something is wrong, contact your child's teacher(s) immediately for an appointment.
- Whenever you do meet with school officials, choose a time when you don't have to rush off to another meeting or engagement. Give yourself time to communicate clearly and without time pressures. Be prepared to ask questions, and bring along a notepad to take notes if needed.

Children who need to take short rest periods or brief breaks to do relaxation exercises should understand that such requests are not ways to avoid class or schoolwork. Any work missed will need to be done later. Parents should emphasize that taking such breaks and maintaining school work are very positive steps, not signs of weakness, and that they give children some control over their pain rather than allowing it to control them.

BOTTOM LINE

The important thing to remember from this chapter is that your child should be involved as much as possible in making decisions about how he will thrive in the world. Your role is to offer suggestions, provide guidance, and then step back to a degree that is appropriate for your child's age and understanding. Rather than curtail your child's leisure and social activities, work along with your child to modify them to fit his or her current level of functioning. The same approach can be taken in regards to your child's education. When there is a team effort—healthcare practitioners, school personnel, you, and your child—steps can be taken that will allow your child to thrive in the school environment as well.

Part III

Bringing Back the Laughter

Chapter 9

PARENTS ASK QUESTIONS ABOUT CHILDHOOD PAIN

What's the difference between acute and chronic pain?

Acute pain, whether it's mild or severe, or whether it lasts a few minutes or a few days, is pain that has an identifiable cause and that goes away as the body heals. Examples of acute pain include stubbing your toe, having your tonsils removed, and burning your hand on a stove. In acute pain, you can usually take some form of medication, such as aspirin or ibuprofen or codeine, or apply an ointment to a burn or cut, and the pain is relieved.

By definition, chronic pain is pain that persists for more than three months. In chronic pain, the cause cannot be removed or taken out of the body. That's because the pain signals keep firing, triggering the nervous system for weeks, months, and even years. Sometimes the cause of the pain is identifiable, such as in juvenile rheumatoid arthritis, in which joint inflammation is involved in the pain process. In other cases, such as complex regional pain syndrome (CRPS), the cause of the pain is unknown. Chronic pain may be continuous or appear as flare-ups and, if untreated, can have a significantly negative effect on people's lives. Children who experience chronic pain often find it difficult to concentrate in school, get adequate sleep, and socialize with friends and family. Living with chronic pain can lead to depression, frustration, anxiety, and feelings of hopelessness. Fortunately, with proper treatment, both the physical and emotional pain can be managed effectively.

How is childhood chronic pain different from chronic pain that adults experience?

We cover this question in detail in Chapter 1, but the brief answer is that there are several significant ways they differ. One is that children experience a greater diversity of chronic pain than adults. Whereas most chronic pain in adults is associated with the lower back, children are prone to chronic abdominal pain, migraine, and pain in their limbs (usually complex regional pain syndrome), as well as conditions that typically are first diagnosed during childhood, such as sickle cell anemia, cystic fibrosis, and juvenile rheumatoid arthritis, as well as conditions such as fibromyalgia, irritable bowel syndrome, and childhood cancers.

Two, children express their pain differently. Very young children can't even verbalize their pain, while slightly older children don't have the vocabulary or frame of reference to explain it. Children also lack the ability to understand the cause and the meaning of their pain, which leads to misconceptions and anxiety that amplify the feeling of pain.

Three, children respond differently to pain medications as well as to mind-body pain-relief techniques. When it comes to drugs, infants and children have some biological factors that differ from adults that impact how they respond to medications. And when we consider mind-body therapies, children tend to be more receptive to certain approaches, especially those that use the imagination (e.g., biofeedback, self-hypnosis, guided imagery). They also have little or no preconceived idea about complementary therapies, which usually makes them more willing to try them.

Yet another difference is less direct: children have parents who are nearly always involved in the day-to-day care and management of their child's pain. That makes parents advocates for their children, and as you've seen in examples throughout the book, parental involvement can have both a positive and negative (though unintentional) impact on a child's struggle with chronic pain.

Do infants really feel pain? I understand they used to perform circumcisions or even surgery on infants without the use of painkillers.

This may sound like a ridiculous question, but as recently as the late 1980s and early 1990s, most people—and that includes many health-care practitioners—thought that infants either felt no pain, or did not remember it once it took place. Whenever an infant reacted to a seemingly painful (to adults) situation, such as a slap or a cut, by crying or grimacing, the belief was that these were signs of fear, not pain. Some research indicated that a newborn's pain sensing system was not fully developed and that it included fewer nerves and pain receptor cells than children and adults. It was also thought that the use of strong painkillers could cause an infant to stop breathing unless he or she was monitored very closely. Thus, male infants were routinely circumcised without the use of pain medication, and because of concerns about giving anesthetics to infants, many babies underwent surgery without receiving painkillers.

We now know that babies feel pain. In fact, experts in fetal development believe that the nerve pathways in a twenty-nine-week-old fetus are functional and capable of transmitting pain signals from the body to the brain.

Not only do fetuses and infants feel pain, but the pain they experience is believed to have a significant, perhaps even a lifelong impact on them. According to Dr. Kanwaljeet J. Anand, a pain and critical care specialist at Arkansas Children's Hospital, premature infants who undergo repetitive painful procedures may be at risk of developing learning delays once they reach school age. His research suggested that behavior problems, difficulties with memory, attention deficit, and learning disabilities could be associated with such pain. It has also been demonstrated that infant boys who are circumcised without local anesthetics respond more vigorously to later painful events in infancy, such as immunizations, than boys who were circumcised with local anesthetics. In other words, even though the infants cannot tell us about their memory of circumcision, the pain of that event affects their behavior for many months to come.

My nine-year-old son was having severe headaches for weeks before he said anything to us. Why would he keep it a secret? It's a myth that children will tell you if they are in pain. Children have an incredible ability to adapt, and so they may not show visible signs of pain. Instead, often they become introspective, quiet, moody, and depressed and try to cope with it on their own. Parents who notice any of these signs should ask their child if he or she is experiencing any type of pain.

How old should a child be before a parent tries to explain why he or she has chronic pain? My son is only four years

old and was recently diagnosed with juvenile rheumatoid arthritis.

At four years old, most children can understand a simple explanation of why they have pain. If you look at Bobbie's story in Chapter 7, you can see an example of how to explain a chronic pain condition to a young child. There are also several other options: (1) You may find it helpful to get some books that are written for children about your child's specific condition (see the Appendix) and either read them with the child or read them yourself and then use their explanation as a guide; (2) ask your health-care practitioner or a child life specialist to help you with the explanation; (3) contact the appropriate organization (e.g., the Arthritis Foundation if you want information about juvenile rheumatoid arthritis) for literature, videos, or other materials and/or someone who can help you discuss your child's condition.

My teenage daughter has sickle cell anemia. She has several crises a year, and she misses school every time. Now she's having trouble fitting in with the kids at her high school. How can I help her feel more accepted?

Sickle cell anemia can be troubling for a young woman as she becomes an adolescent. Along with all the pressures that come with the teenage years—hormone changes, dating, peer acceptance, keeping up grades—the challenges of sickle cell disease can be overwhelming. Often teenagers feel isolated from their friends because they feel they are "different" or "strange," and that no one will understand. And most normal teenagers want to be like all the other teenagers in their peer group more than anything else. Being "different" is a curse to the average teen.

Several things may help your daughter feel more accepted. One is talking with a psychologist who can help her with coping skills and issues of self-esteem. Another is to find other teens who also have sickle cell so she can share her experiences and feelings with them. If you can't find a local support group, there are online chats, such as the one sponsored by the American Sickle Cell Anemia Association (see Appendix). It would also help if your daughter could establish a close relationship with another teen who is supportive and who understands the challenges your daughter faces. You should talk to your daughter about who that person could be and even offer suggestions, but the final decision must be hers.

My son was diagnosed with juvenile rheumatoid arthritis last year. He's at the age (nine) where all of his friends are playing on Little League and other teams, and the kids are teasing him because he can't participate like they can. How can I help him feel better about himself?

Participating in sports is a dream for many young boys, and for those who have juvenile rheumatoid arthritis, it's one that can offer some significant challenges. One possibility is to talk with the coach of a team your son wants to play on and see if there is an alternative way for him to participate. For example, if he enjoys baseball, perhaps he can be a hitter and have a designated runner. He may shadow one of the coaches and learn about that aspect of the sport.

Switching to another competitive sport that is better for your child's illness is another good option. Swimming is an excellent sport and a great exercise for children who have juvenile rheumatoid arthritis because it doesn't harm the joints. You might suggest to your son that he join a swimming group, where he could also make some new friends who would share his interest.

How should children explain their health problems to their friends?

First, children need to have accurate, clear information about their condition. Then, once they are comfortable with or confident enough to speak about it, they should choose when, how, and whom they will tell. Although you may want to do the explaining for them, your role is to help your child understand the condition, offer help if he or she asks for it, and then let your child have control over the telling.

I'm worried about my son getting constipation from the opioids our doctor just prescribed. How can I prevent it or treat it without drugs?

Constipation is a very common side effect of opioid use, and may also cause other symptoms such as nausea, vomiting, and abdominal cramps. If you want to help prevent constipation or treat it should it occur, without the use of medications, encourage your child to eat foods rich in fiber, such as fruits, vegetables, and whole grains. Foods that children may enjoy include oatmeal with raisins, high-fiber cereals such as Fiber One or Bran Chex, a bean taco made with kidney beans, corn on the cob, and sweet potatoes. He should also drink six to eight eight-ounce glasses of water daily. Moderate activity, if your child is up to it, also helps keep waste moving through the intestinal tract. If a laxative becomes necessary, Senokot, Maalox, and Dulcolax can be used with a doctor's supervision. Dulcolax is available as a suppository, which is helpful if your child is vomiting and can't keep food down.

My ten-year-old daughter suffers with chronic daily headaches and sometimes has to miss school because of it. I was wondering, how common are headaches in school age children?

Your daughter is among the 10 percent of children between the ages of nine and eighteen who suffer with head pain that is sufficient to cause them to miss school, curtail social activities, and disrupt other areas of their lives. Headaches that occur during the school year can be especially upsetting to parents and children for several reasons. It can be difficult to know whether you should insist your child go to school because of fears he or she may fall behind. Some children, especially those who enjoy school and who are doing well, may have the same fears. Staying home from school may not be an option for some parents if, for example, in a single-parent household the parent can't stay home from work and there is no one to watch the child. Children who suffer with chronic or migraine headache may also feel alienated from their friends or need to stop participating in activities that aggravate or trigger head pain, such as sports.

Headaches can affect how well your child functions in school. One study found school-related problems in 46 percent of adolescent headache patients. Another study reported that young headache patients name "school" as the main headache trigger, ahead of parents, lack of sleep, missed meals, and the weather. School children who have headache at school must also deal with school-related noise, bus exhaust, and bright lights, which can exacerbate their pain.

According to the 1989 National Health Interview Survey, children between the ages of seven and seventeen who had chronic daily headache and who were being treated in a pediatric specialty practice missed about fifty-seven days of school per year. About 10 percent of children of the same age who have migraine miss more than two school days per month. In another study, children with recurrent headache reportedly missed 3.3 days per child per year. Obviously there is a wide range in the number of missed school days for children with different types of headache. What's relevant to you, however, is your own child and the effect head pain has on him or her.

When children miss more and more school, their stress levels rise and they fall behind in their schoolwork. They may miss out on school and other social events. Other students may tease them about missing school, and teachers and school officials may question the legitimacy of the headaches. The anxiety associated with these situations may lead the child to not want to return to school to face these pressures, leading to school avoidance behavior patterns. Therefore if your child has chronic headache that affects his or her school attendance and performance, make sure you have your health-care practitioner talk with school officials about your child's needs and a headache treatment plan (see Chapter 8). Once school personnel are aware of the legitimacy of your child's pain, they will be more willing to help your child.

My daughter has juvenile fibromyalgia, and a friend told me that massage would help. Where can I find a qualified massage therapist?

It's true that massage is often recommended as therapy for children who have juvenile fibromyalgia, but before you look for a professional therapist, you should talk with your child's physician and physical therapist to make sure massage is recommended for your child. They may be able to refer you to a qualified individual. If they cannot, or you wish to locate one on your own, you can contact the American Massage Therapy Association or the National Certification Board for Therapeutic Massage and Bodywork (see Appendix) for a qualified practitioner in your area.

Professional massage therapists have credentials that can include CMT (Certified Massage Therapist), LMT (Licensed Massage Therapist), or RMT (Registered Massage Therapist). Make sure the practitioner you choose has experience working with juvenile fibromyalgia.

My doctor thinks my five-year-old son has migraines. Isn't that too young for migraine?

No. Experts believe migraine can occur in children as young as one to two years of age, and perhaps even earlier. One possible early sign of migraine is colic, as it's been shown that a large number of infants who are colicky have migraine in later life. Another possible sign of the tendency to suffer with migraine is moderate to severe motion sickness at an early age. Your doctor may have asked you if your child had any of these symptoms as an infant.

Why did the doctor recommend my eleven-year-old daughter see a psychologist? She has fibromyalgia, she's not crazy!

Your daughter seeing a psychologist has nothing to do with her being "crazy." Chronic and persistent pain is more than physical; it can cause a lot of stress, anxiety, and depression, all of which can make pain worse. While a doctor can help take care of some of the physical pain, a psychologist can also help your child deal with that pain by learning how to use his or her mind. A psychologist can teach your child coping skills, such as relaxation exercises and behavior modification. Some psychologists are also trained to teach self-hypnosis, biofeedback, meditation, and guided imagery, all skills that have been shown to help reduce pain.

Fibromyalgia, like many chronic pain conditions, lasts a lifetime, and so it is important that your daughter learn as many coping skills as possible. A psychologist can help her with that process. Also, chronic pain is a family affair, so it may be helpful at some point if you or other family members also talk with a psychologist about your feelings and how you cope with any stress related to your daughter's condition. Seeing a psychologist should be viewed as just another form of treatment, as is a prescription for a painkiller or a visit with a physical therapist.

My doctor prescribed opioids for my eight-year-old son, who has cancer. Can he become addicted to these drugs?

Although it is true that opioids (narcotics) can lead to addiction in susceptible individuals, it is very rare for children who are being treated with opioids for severe or chronic pain to become addicted. Many people confuse "tolerance" and "physical dependence" with "psychological dependence" and "addiction." Most people, of any age, who take opioids become tolerant of these drugs. That means that over time, they may need to take higher and higher doses to get the same pain-relieving effect. Tolerance is a normal physiological response to the use of opioids. Physical dependence is defined as the development of withdrawal symptoms when someone suddenly stops taking opioids. Symptoms may include muscle aches, sweating, diarrhea, and irritability. Like tolerance, these symptoms are a normal physiological response when someone who has been taking opioids for two weeks or longer abruptly stops taking them. Withdrawal symptoms can be avoided if the individual gradually reduces the dose over several days to two weeks, preferably with a doctor's guidance.

Psychological dependence, or addiction, is defined as compulsive drug use characterized by a continued craving for the drug and a need to take the drug for effects other than pain relief. Less than 1 percent of patients who take opioids for pain control under medical supervision ever become addicted to their medication. Therefore, you should not be concerned that your child will become addicted.

Why are antidepressants and antiseizure drugs used to treat chronic pain?

Experts have found that the chemicals the body uses to block or send pain messages (e.g., serotonin) are the same as those that become out of balance when a person is depressed. Some chronic pain conditions are caused by nerves that fire in ways and at times that are inappropriate, which is similar to what occurs when someone has a seizure. Researchers have discovered that while antidepressants and antiseizure drugs are effective in treating the conditions for which they were developed, they also often provide a side benefit—pain relief. In addition, antidepressants and antiseizure drugs also improve mood and help with sleep, both of which have an effect on pain. See Chapter 6 for more information on these and other types of drugs that are used to treat pain.

When should I consider taking my child to a pediatric pain clinic? Our pediatrician has been treating my daughter for migraine and chronic headache for about six months, and we haven't seen much improvement with the treatment she has been receiving.

Any time you are uncertain or displeased with your child's treatment, you should first talk with the doctor and express your concerns. The doctor may then refer you to a pediatric pain clinic or a specialist. Even if the doctor does not refer you, however, you can still seek a clinic on your own (see Appendix). While pediatricians can handle many pain complaints quite well, pain that doesn't respond to standard treatment or that can be more complicated in nature, such as complex regional pain syndrome, cancer pain, endometriosis, and arthritis-type pain, may require more specialty care, such as that found in pediatric pain clinics.

Our doctor said our child should be involved in her own pain management, but she's only nine years old. What can she do?

Children as young as three and four can have some say in their pain management. For example, a four-year-old who needs to take a certain medication that comes only in oral form can be asked if he wants to take it with chocolate pudding or applesauce. A three-year-old who needs to have a blood sample taken can be asked which finger the nurse can prick. Notice that the four-year-old isn't given the option of taking or not taking the medication, just *how* he will take it. Similarly, the three-year-old isn't asked *if* he wants his finger pricked, just which one. A fourteen-year-old, however, can be told about the possible side effects of a specific pain medication and then decide if he or she wants to take the drug and risk side effects or decline the medication.

A nine-year-old child can make choices about the type of coping skills she wants to use. For example, her doctor may explain how self-hypnosis, biofeedback, guided imagery, breathing exercises, and relaxation exercises work and she can decide which ones she wants to learn. Involvement in pain management can also include how much information your child wants about her condition or about a procedure. Children who need to have blood drawn or an intravenous needle inserted should be asked if they want to know how the procedure will be done and also told they can choose to watch or not watch. When children are allowed to participate in their pain management, even in small ways, it gives them a sense of control over the situation and helps build self-confidence.

Pain is a very subjective and personal experience, and only your child knows how much pain she or he is experiencing. Therefore, you need to trust when your child says he or she is feeling pain or that a specific procedure is painful, unless you have good reason not to believe it. Remember, however, that the anticipation of pain and the fear and anxiety that go along with it, as in when a child may need to undergo a spinal tap or even the drawing of blood, can be very real to a child. If you think your child is reacting to the fear and not to pain from a physical cause, then you and the health-care practitioner can defuse the fear by using various distraction techniques (see Chapter 4).

I have had endometriosis since my early twenties, and now my fifteen-year-old daughter has been diagnosed with it as well. Can endometriosis be inherited?

Several studies show that there is almost an eightfold increase in the risk of developing endometriosis in women whose mother or sister has the disease. One of the studies that included more than 150 women with endometriosis showed that 12 percent had a mother or sister with the disease, while only 1.5 percent had a mother-in-law or sister-in-law with endometriosis. Researchers also found that women who had a family history of endometriosis tended to have a more aggressive form of the disease.

My daughter was recently diagnosed with fibromyalgia, and her doctor told us there's no medication for this disease. Is that true?

It's true that there are no medications to specifically treat fibromyalgia, but there are several ways to treat the symptoms effectively and to improve the quality of your child's life. One way to battle her fatigue is to prescribe medication to improve her sleep. It's critical that she get an adequate amount of sleep every night—eight to nine hours—and that she maintain a regular sleep pattern by going to bed at around the same time every night. She should also make sure she does stretching exercises daily and also does some sort of aerobic activity, such as walking or bicycling every day. Her exercise program should be developed and monitored by a physical therapist to make sure she gets an adequate amount of exercise but doesn't overexert herself. Stress management techniques, such as relaxation exercises, deep breathing, meditation, and yoga, are also recommended.

There are a lot of over-the-counter drugs on the market for pain. Which ones are safe for an eight-year-old child? My son frequently has severe headaches.

If your child has frequent, severe headache, you should have a pediatrician examine him. Any headache that lasts for more than five days in a child also requires a doctor's visit. The younger the child, the more critical it is to see a doctor if your child suffers with headache. That being said, there are some cautions to consider before you give your child a nonprescription medication. Naturally, I recommend you talk to your pediatrician before you give your child any type of medication, including herbal formulas.

Most nonprescription drugs have warnings against their use in younger children. Acetaminophen (Tylenol), for example, should not be given to children younger than two years unless your doctor gives you specific instructions. Aspirin should *never* be given to a child younger than sixteen years of age because of the risk of Reye's syndrome (see Chapter 6). Ibuprofen is considered a safe drug for children, and it comes in different formulas for different ages, although there are no formulations for children younger than six months. Several ibuprofen products come as a liquid oral suspension and concentrated drops, which can be used in children as young as two years. Naproxen sodium (Aleve) should not be given to children younger than age twelve, and ketoprofen (Orudis KT) should not be used in children younger than age sixteen.

In all cases, you should read the label carefully to see how long you can treat your child before a visit to your pediatrician is recommended and/or you should discontinue use of the drug. For some drugs, the allowed time is as short as forty-eight hours.

Are there any effective topical medications for pain?

There are several safe and effective ointments, creams, or gels that can be used to relieve minor pain associated with fibromyalgia, juvenile rheumatoid arthritis, and other muscle or joint pain. These medications can be helpful for enhancing the pain-killing effects of other medications your child may be taking.

One topical medication is capsaicin (Zostrix, Capzasin-P, and others), a natural ingredient found in hot chili peppers. Capsaicin works by depleting the substance that relays pain—substance P—to the brain from the nerve endings in the skin. It is also available in a patch (TheraPatch) and roll-on stick. Some people experience a burning sensation or itching when they use these products, and that limits their effectiveness in children. However, if they can tolerate the burning for a few days, it ultimately stops while the analgesic effect continues.

There are also substances such as camphor, eucalyptus oil, oil of wintergreen, and menthol, which create a feeling of heat or cold when they are applied to the hurting area. Brands include ArthriCare, Eucalyptamint, Icy Hot, Menthacin (which also includes capsaicin), and Therapeutic Mineral Ice.

Yet another category are salicylates, substances that reduce pain and inflammation by seeping through the skin. Brands include Aspercreme, BenGay, Flexall, and Sportscreme.

My three-year-old gets very upset when he needs to get a needle or have blood drawn. What can I or the doctor do to reduce the pain associated with minor medical procedures?

Much of the response you see in children who need to undergo minor medical procedures, such as needlesticks or blood draws, or even more complicated procedures such as bone marrow aspiration and lumbar punctures is associated with their anticipation of the event. You can help take the "sting" out of their anticipation by doing the following:

- Ask a health-care professional about how the procedure works, how it feels, and how long it will last.
- Explain the procedure to your child, including where it will be done, who will do it, how it will help him or her, and how long it will take, using simple language. Be honest about the procedure; let your child know what may hurt and what won't hurt.
- Use "non-scary" language in your explanation. For example, if your child needs an injection of a contrast substance, use the word "medicine" instead of "dye." Instead of the phrase "put you to sleep," say "make you tired" or "make you dream."
- Stay with your child during the procedure if possible. Offer comfort if needed, such as holding a hand, hugging, or letting your child sit on your lap.
- Let your child know that many children have the procedure. It's important that your child know that having this procedure isn't a punishment.
- Ask your child if he or she has any questions and encourage sharing.
- Let your child have a role in the procedure (if possible). For example, he or she may choose which finger will be used for a needlestick.
- Practice coping strategies, such as deep breathing or guided imagery. Distraction is often effective (see Chapter 4), such blowing bubbles, singing, reading a favorite story, or watching a video.

Health-care practitioners have several topical products that also can take the sting out of these procedures. One is lidocaine, which is available in a patch (Lidoderm) or cream (Elemax). Once the lidocaine is applied to the area of the body to be treated, it numbs the area for up to 150 minutes. Elemax is available over the counter from pharmacies, and can be applied one-half hour before needle puncture to reduce or eliminate the pain of this event.

Chapter 10

STORIES OF SUCCESS

When you think about chronic pain, what is your definition of "success"? As parents, I'm sure you want to define it as "complete elimination of pain," but in the real world, this is usually not the case. But we can improve the pain: we can make it manageable, we can give children some control over it, and we can improve the quality of their lives. Even with the worst cases, we can still make a significant, positive difference.

Achieving that difference doesn't come without some hard work on the part of the children and their parents, hard work in the form of working closely with all the health-care practitioners—physician, physical and/or occupational therapist, psychologist, and perhaps other specialists; regularly practicing coping skills; sticking with the programs developed by the physical and/or occupational therapist; being willing to try new therapies; seeking help from support groups and appropriate organizations; and maintaining a pain diary when one is recommended.

I have already shared many stories with you throughout this book. Some of the cases were very challenging; others reached a satisfactory conclusion within a much shorter time. In this chapter I bring you several more stories, two told in the words of the children themselves, and two through the eyes of their parents. As in the previous chapters, I hope something within these stories will strike a chord, offer you hope, provide information you didn't have before, and give you ideas for new directions you and your child can take. Remember, you are not alone. Millions of children and families share your plight. There is hope for every child who suffers with chronic pain.

MICHELLE'S STORY

"When I was fifteen, I was bowling with some friends on a Saturday morning when one of them dropped a bowling ball on my right foot. It really hurt at first, but I didn't think I had broken anything so we stayed and kept bowling a few games. Later that night, however, the bottom of my foot started to burn, which I thought was weird because the ball had hit the top of my foot. My foot kept burning for a few days, but I could walk on it. When I woke up Thursday morning, my foot was red and swollen, the skin was a lot colder than my left foot, and the burning was now on top of my foot. The worst part was, when I stepped out of bed, I fell down because the pain was so bad I couldn't stand on my foot.

"My dad took me to the emergency room and they took X-rays, but nothing was broken. The emergency room doctor referred us to a neurologist, who told me I might have CRPS. I didn't even know what that was, and after the doctor explained it, all I wanted to know was when it would go away. He said he didn't know and gave me two prescriptions—one for amitriptyline and another for verapamil—and said they would help the pain.

"Well, they didn't. For a week, the pain got worse, and it even spread to my ankle. I couldn't stand to wear a sock or even have anyone touch my foot, it hurt so bad. On a scale of 1 to 10, the pain was definitely an 8 to 10 most of the time. We went back to the neurologist, and he prescribed lidocaine transdermal patches and scheduled me for physical therapy three times a week, but the lidocaine didn't help enough for me to get through the therapy.

"That's when the doctor decided to refer us to a pain management clinic. The pain management team there told me they were going to do something called a sympathetic nerve block, and they did two of them, but they didn't help except for only a day or two.

"By this time I was getting really angry because I was supposed to start tenth grade in a few weeks, and I was supposed to be on the soccer team, and I couldn't even walk. Next the doctors took me off the amitryptiline and gave me gabapentin. They also told me to keep my foot in a whirlpool at home, and that helped while the foot was in the water but not when I had to take it out. That's when the doctors decided to put me in the hospital and do an epidural block, which they kept in for five days. Finally, the pain was so much better, like a 3 out of 10. Even though I was on crutches, I figured I could at least go to school. The first few days of school were great, and my foot hardly hurt at all. I was thinking about the soccer team.

"Then everything fell apart. The pain came back at around an 8, and I had to go back to the hospital. They did another epidural, but it didn't work. I was really scared, and the doctor recommended that I see a psychologist, which I didn't want to do, but he talked me into it because I didn't want to be like this forever.

"By this time I was in a wheelchair because the pain was so bad. I couldn't even go to school. The doctors then prescribed oxycodone, but all it did was make me constipated without relieving my pain, so I stopped taking it. I was so miserable, and my parents were really worried. They decided to take me to another hospital, this time one that specialized in treating children.

"This hospitalization was really different. Instead of epidurals and nerve blocks, they started me on physical and occupational therapy, about four hours a day. They also taught me self-hypnosis, biofeedback, and distraction therapy. I was out of my wheelchair within a few days, and didn't even need the crutches after a week. My foot still hurt, but only about a 2 out of 10. After a month of therapy, I felt great. The doctors took me off all my medications, and I went back to school without crutches. Whenever the pain comes back, and it does every few months, I use self-hypnosis, biofeedback, and the whirlpool to get rid of it, and it works. I decided not to go out for soccer, however, and instead joined the drama team."

WYATT'S STORY

"Our son, Wyatt, was seven when he was diagnosed with juvenile rheumatoid arthritis," says Eve. "My husband, Jeff, and I had taken Wyatt on a camping trip to Colorado in June. Wyatt was so excited because it would be the first time he would help pitch a tent and then go hiking in the mountains. We went hiking every day, not too far each day, and he just loved it. When we got back home to Chicago, he complained that his knee hurt. We thought perhaps he had overdone the hiking a bit, although he hadn't said anything while we were in Colorado. We waited a few days to see if the pain got any better, and in the meantime, one night he got a fever of 103 degrees. We put him to bed immediately and gave him lots of fluids, and in the morning the fever was gone.

"That's when it got strange," says Jeff. "Wyatt was fine the next day, but at night, he got a fever again, and this time he had chills. He also said his knee hurt really bad. We made an appointment with his pediatrician and saw him two days later. The doctor seemed to think that Wyatt had a virus and that with rest, plenty of fluids, and some ibuprofen, he should be fine in a few days."

"But he wasn't," says Eve. "The fevers, chills, and pain continued for another four to five days, so we went back to the doctor, who then consulted with a colleague and referred us to a pediatric rheumatologist. He examined Wyatt, ran a few tests, and told us our son had juvenile rheumatoid arthritis."

Even though it wasn't what Eve and Jeff wanted to hear, they were glad to get a diagnosis so quickly so Wyatt could start with therapy right away. "We knew this was going to be really hard for Wyatt, because he's such an active kid," says Eve. "The first thing he asked the doctor was, 'when can I play baseball again?' The doctor was very diplomatic and told Wyatt that if he worked hard and did what he was told, he could probably be part of the team. He then explained to Wyatt that they may not be able to make the pain go away completely, but that he could learn some ways to make it better.

"Wyatt was started on a physical therapy program that included hydrotherapy and swimming three times a week. The swimming is great for Wyatt, because it's fun. We also considered acupuncture, but Wyatt couldn't be convinced to try it, so Jeff and I learned how to do massage. We massage Wyatt's legs every night for about twenty minutes, and it helps a lot. He's also on a few medications, including methotrexate, which helps delay progression of the disease, and is tolerating it okay.

"I guess the hardest part is making sure Wyatt doesn't overexert himself, yet not prevent him from having fun too," says Eve. "The doctor recommended we keep a diary of Wyatt's activities, medication use, and symptoms so we could make sure we are on track with his treatment. We know that if Wyatt is fairly active one day, he'll need a few days to rest, so we try to keep it in balance. And when his condition flares up, he practices his relaxation exercises and finds things to do in the house. Fortunately, Wyatt has a good friend who likes to trade baseball cards, so they can spend hours doing that when Wyatt isn't able to go out and play."

Eve and Jeff had some concerns about how Wyatt would adjust to school and were even considering home schooling until their doctor and psychologist explained that keeping Wyatt's schedule as normal as possible would be best for him.

"Wyatt was diagnosed about a month before school started, so the whole experience was new to us when it came time for him to go back," says Eve. "We were so grateful when our doctor and the psychologist sat down with us to discuss our concerns about Wyatt. We talked about what his challenges would be, like not being able to participate in recess very much or not at all on some days, that getting around the hallways might be hard when they were crowded, the need to take medications during the day, and needing time off to go to physical therapy three times a week.

"Our doctor called the school nurse, and Jeff and I met with Wyatt's principal, classroom teachers, and the school nurse about his needs. Everyone was very understanding. Wyatt has to change classrooms once a day, and he is allowed to leave a few minutes early so he can avoid the crowded halls. His medication is being handled by the school nurse, and we scheduled his physical therapy sessions so he misses a minimum of school, and any work he misses he takes home. Recess is still a bit of a problem. We don't want to prevent him from playing with his friends, but he tries to keep up with them, and then he's in a lot of pain the next few days. His teacher tries to limit his activities the best she can. It's all a learning process for all of us right now."

Eve and Jeff have found an arthritis support group, and they meet with other parents of children who have juvenile arthritis. "Getting together with other parents and children has helped us and Wyatt a great deal," says Jeff. "Wyatt has met other kids just like him, and he doesn't feel out of place when he's around them. There's even a camp for children with arthritis, and we're going to send Wyatt there next summer."

"We know our son has many challenges ahead of him," says Eve. "But we're happy with the help we've gotten from the medical staff, the school, and our support group, and I think we're going to be okay."

SIERRA'S STORY

"I remember thinking, 'this can't be normal, this can't be what women go through each month.' I remember I just wanted to die, the pain was so bad. And I remember the school nurse telling me, 'every woman gets cramps, and you'll get used to it.' But I never did."

Sierra, who was fourteen when she first experienced the pain of endometriosis, is now a freshman in college. She looks back at the first five years of her life with endometriosis and the path she took to where she is today.

"I started to menstruate just a few weeks before my fourteenth birthday," says Sierra. "I knew something was going on about a week before it happened, because I was feeling bloated and crampy. A few of my friends already had their periods, and none of them said the pain was a big deal. In fact, my first few cycles weren't too bad, but I did take ibuprofen for a few days each time.

"I think it was my fourth or fifth period that was really terrible. I was doubled over with pain, and I couldn't go to school for four days. I know my mother believed me when I said the pain was unbearable, because I really liked school and was very involved with the drama club and the drill team. We both thought that that time was just a fluke, but it wasn't. After that one time, my periods were agony. I remember I had a big part in a musical at school, and on the first night of the performance, I had such horrible cramps I couldn't even stand up straight. An understudy played my part, and I was furious.

"My friends didn't understand how my periods could be so painful, and thought I had found a way to get out of going to school three or four days a month. But I wasn't just missing school; I also had to drop out of the drill team because I couldn't make all the practices and games, and I quit the drama club because I could never be sure the pain wouldn't prevent me from performing again.

"Fortunately, my mother believed me and insisted I go to a gynecologist. By that time, I had been having pain for nearly a year. Each month, the pain would start about four days before my menstrual flow and continue for another three to four days. During that time I couldn't sleep, and during the worst pain I kept a heating pad on my stomach most of the time.

"The gynecologist diagnosed me as having primary dysmenorrhea (painful menstruation) and prescribed birth control pills. After taking them for two months, I didn't feel any better. Then she prescribed acetaminophen with codeine, which took the edge off the pain but also made me too drowsy to function in school. So now I was falling asleep in class, and still had a lot of pain.

"In the meantime, my mother read something about endometriosis and asked the gynecologist to test me for it. When I found out I needed to undergo laparoscopic surgery, I said I didn't want to do it. It only took one more agonizing few days around my next period to convince me that I should give it a try. The surgery was scheduled for two weeks after my period.

"When the surgery was over and the doctor told us that she didn't find any evidence of endometriosis, I started to worry there was something else terribly serious wrong with me. My mother told the doctor she didn't believe her, and by the time I got home from the hospital, my mother said she had found another alternative: a pain management hospital.

"I wasn't too keen on the idea, but after we talked about it, I decided to go. I saw Dr. Krane, and after an extensive interview and examination, he recommended I have another laparoscopy, but this time when I was experiencing pain. He also suggested something the other doctor had not: some alternative ways to treat and deal with the pain, like acupuncture, self-hypnosis, exercise, and meditation, and some sessions with a psychologist.

"At first I agreed to try anything and everything, because I didn't want to go through high school that way any more. The second laparoscopy did show endometriosis, and the surgeon removed the adhesions. Immediately after the surgery I started seeing the psychologist and learning self-hypnosis and meditation. I met with a physical therapist, who showed me some yoga poses and said I needed to do brisk walking or swimming—whichever was most comfortable at the time—at least five times a week.

"Two weeks after the surgery I got my period and the pain returned, but this time it was less severe. I had changed my mind about the acupuncture and thought I'd wait to see how the surgery, self-hypnosis, and exercise worked. I was still taking birth control pills, but I had stopped the acetaminophen with codeine.

"I soon grew frustrated with self-hypnosis and meditation, so about two months after the surgery, I decided to go for the acupuncture. I started treatments twice a week. To tell the truth, I wasn't expecting much from them, and was actually nervous about the needles. But the acupuncturist was very gentle, and all I ever felt was twinges when the needles were placed.

"After two weeks of treatment, I got my period—and it was nearly pain free. I was so excited I couldn't believe it. I continued with two more weeks of acupuncture treatments, and then went back for a 'refresher' treatment about once a month for a year.

"That was two years ago, and now my periods are fairly normal—just regular cramps. I know the endometriosis can come back at any time, but if it does, I'm prepared to deal with it."

SHAWN'S STORY

"Our son, Shawn, was eight years old, and had been suffering with migraines and chronic daily headache for more than two years before we saw Dr. Krane," says Lisa. "Up until that time, I felt as though we had exhausted every avenue to find a way to help our son. We had been to two pediatricians, a neurologist, and a naturopath. Shawn had had MRI scans, X-rays, and allergy tests, and the only thing the doctors found was hay fever; otherwise he was in good health.

"In the beginning, Shawn was getting three migraines a month," explains Lisa, "each one lasting for a few hours, with nausea and vomiting, and then he would sleep for several hours and wake up nearly pain free. That's when the first doctor we saw put Shawn on daily propranolol for his chronic daily headaches and another prescription for sumatriptan (Imitrex) spray to stop migraine attacks. After a few months, Shawn wasn't getting any better, and that's when a friend suggested we see a naturopath. She suggested we eliminate sugars and nitrates from Shawn's diet and to get him to eat more whole foods, organic if possible."

Changing Shawn's diet was difficult at first, but Lisa and her husband, David, decided they would make the same changes to their diet so Shawn wouldn't feel he was being punished. They also knew that it was basically a healthier way to eat, and because Shawn tended to be a little heavy, they also hoped it would help keep his weight in check.

"Two months after we made the dietary changes, we did see some improvement," says Lisa. "Shawn was now getting an average of two migraines per month and the daily headaches were somewhat less severe. But we still felt we had a long way to go.

"We then went to another doctor, who examined Shawn and referred us to a neurologist. The neurologist tapered Shawn off the propranolol and started him on cyproheptadine (Periactin), but kept him on sumatriptan. As it was nearly time for school to start, we hoped this new treatment plan would help keep him from missing school. I even think Shawn was optimistic at first, but after two months of no change in the frequency of the migraines and the severity of his daily headaches, we began to feel frustrated. To make things worse, Shawn was gaining too much weight, even on the healthier eating plan, and we learned that cyproheptadine was probably the cause. We were ready to find a new doctor, and that's when a relative told us about Lucile Packard Children's Hospital.

"We were very impressed by the treatment we got at the hospital," says Lisa. "Shawn got the most intensive examination ever, and David and I were questioned about every aspect of our son's life, including his eating and sleeping habits, moods, schoolwork, friends, play activities, medication use, and medical history. No one had ever bothered to ask so many questions before. One thing we said that really struck a chord with the doctor was that Shawn tends to be a perfectionist and to get angry with himself if he doesn't 'get it right,' whether it's his schoolwork, playing a game, making a model, or playing sports. However, we have never pushed him to do things he didn't want to do, like insist he play Little League or take piano lessons.

"By the end of our first meeting with Dr. Krane, we walked out of the hospital with a plan, but quite honestly, not the plan I had had in mind originally. I thought he would just change Shawn's medication, but instead we had an appointment for Shawn and us to see a child psychologist (at separate times), we were shown how to keep a daily pain diary for the next three weeks, and we talked about coping skills for Shawn to learn. And, oh yes, Dr. Krane did begin to taper Shawn off the cyproheptadine, which was causing weight gain and not providing much relief, and started him on nortriptyline.

"The psychologist immediately began to teach Shawn coping skills, including breathing exercises, progressive relaxation, and self-hypnosis. Shawn was excited about the self-hypnosis, and he learned it easily. These are skills Shawn can use at home as well as at school, so we were pleased, too, because we hoped they would help Shawn not miss much school.

"During our visit with the psychologist, we learned that we needed to keep Shawn's life as normal as possible, to encourage him to use his coping skills whenever he felt a migraine coming on or to deal with his chronic headaches, and to keep up with the diary so we could monitor Shawn's pain as well as his medication use and responses to it.

"David and I were most impressed with the coping skills Shawn was shown," says Lisa. "None of the other doctors had ever pointed out the huge role stress plays in migraines and chronic headaches. Of course, it makes sense to us now, but it wasn't until Dr. Krane and the psychologist explained it to us and then gave Shawn some real ways to deal with it that we realized just how important this type of treatment can be.

"Today, Shawn is ten years old going on thirty," says Lisa. "I truly think his experiences with migraine and daily headaches and all the health-care professionals have made him mature faster than other kids his age. He still gets migraines, but only about one every other month, and these he treats immediately with sumatriptan spray. His chronic headaches haven't disappeared either, but they only come about once a week. We keep after Shawn to practice his coping skills daily, even though he doesn't get headaches as often as he used to, but he's come to realize that he needs to do his exercises in order to stay as headache-free as possible."

Appendix

RELEVANT READING

American Society of Anesthesiologists. Acupuncture no child's play: it helps get kids better. News release, October 15, 2002.

Arthritis Foundation, ed. *Raising a Child with Arthritis: Parent's Guide.* National Book Network, 1998.

Ball, T.M., D.E. Shapiro, C.J. Monheim, and J.A. Weydert. A pilot study of use of guided imagery for treatment of recurrent abdominal pain in children. *Clin Pediatr (Phil)* 2003 Jul–Aug; 42(6): 527–32.

Ballweg, Mary Lou, and the Endometriosis Association. *Endometriosis: The Complete Reference for Taking Charge of Your Health.* Chicago/New York: Contemporary Books, 2004.

Brandes, J.L., et al. Topiramate for migraine prevention. *JAMA* 2004; 291(8): 965–73.

Brown, C.R. Pain management. Biofeedback and relaxation therapy. *Pract Periodontics Aesthet Dent* 1997; 9: 1068.

Chabal, C., D.A. Fishbain, M. Weaver, and L.W. Heine. Long-term transcutaneous electrical nerve stimulation (TENS) use: Impact on medication utilization and physical therapy costs. *Clin J Pain* 1998; 14: 66–73.

Chalkiadis, G.A. Management of chronic pain in children. *Med J Aust* 2001; 175: 476–79.

Cheyette, Sarah, M.D. *Mommy, My Head Hurts.* Newmarket Press, 2002.

Collins, J.J., et al. Transdermal fentanyl in children with cancer pain: Feasibility, tolerability, and pharmacokinetic correlates. *J Pediatr* 1999; 134: 319–23.

Conte, P.M., G.A. Walco, and Y. Kimura. Temperament and stress response in children with juvenile primary fibromyalgia syndrome. *Arthris Rheum* 2003 Oct; 48(10): 2923–30.

Crushell, E., et al. Importance of parental conceptual model of illness in severe recurrent abdominal pain. *Pediatrics* 2003; 112: 1368–72.

Diamond, Seymour, and Amy Diamond. *Headache and Your Child: The Complete Guide to Understanding and Treating Migraine and Other Headaches in Children and Adolescents.* New York: Fireside, 2001.

Dinges, D.F., W.G. Whitehouse, E.C. Orne, P.B. Bloom, M.M. Carlin, N.K. Bauer, K.A. Gillen, B.S. Shapiro, K. Ohene-Frempong, C. Dampier, and M.T. Orne. Self-hypnosis training as an adjunctive treatment in the management of pain associated with sickle cell disease. *Int J Clin Exp Hypn* 1997 Oct; 45(4): 417–32.

Ferrari, M.D., et al. Oral triptans in acute migraine treatment: A meta-analysis of 53 trials. *Lancet* 2001; 358: 1668–75.

Field, T., M. Hernandez-Reif, S. Seligman, J. Krasnegor, W. Sunshine, R. Rivas-Chacon, S. Schanberg, and C. Kuhn. Juvenile rheumatoid arthritis: Benefits from massage therapy. *J Pediatr Psycho* 1997 Oct; 22(5): 607–17.

Gil, K.M., et al. Daily coping practice predicts treatment effects in children with sickle cell disease. *J Pediatric Psychology* 2001; 26(3): 163–73.

Jacobson, A. ASA: Acupuncture dramatically reduces pain in pediatric pain management clinic. *Doctors Group News,* October 17, 2002.

Kemper, K.J., et al. On pins and needles? Pediatric pain patients' experience with acupuncture. *Pediatrics* 2000; 105: 941–47.

Koseoglu, E., et al. Aerobic exercise and plasma beta endorphin levels in patients with migrainous headache without aura. *Cephalalgia* 2003; 23: 972–76.

Laufer, M.R., J. Sanfilippo, and G. Rose. Adolescent endometriosis: Diagnosis and treatment approaches. *J Pediatr Adolsc Gynecol* 2003 Jun; 16(3Suppl): S3–11.

Lin, Y.C., et al. Pediatric medial acupuncture service. Presented at the 55th Annual Meeting of the American Society of Anesthesiologists, Orlando, FL, October 16, 2002. Abstract A-1293.

Loewy, Joanne V., ed. *Music Therapy and Pediatric Pain.* Cherry Hill, NJ: Jeffrey Books, 1997.

McGrath, P.A. Development of the World Health Organization Guidelines on Cancer Pain Relief and Palliative Care in Children. *J Pain Symptom Manage* 1995; 12: 87–92.

Mellick, G.A., and L.B. Mellick. Reflex sympathetic dystrophy treated with gabapentin. *Arch Phys Med Rehabil* 1997; 78: 98–105.

Montgomery, G.H., K.N. DuHamel, and W.H. Redd. A meta-analysis of hypnotically induced analgesia: How effective is hypnosis? *Int J Clin Exp Hypn* 2000; 48: 138–53.

O'Hara, Mary Jo, R.N., et al. Pain management in children with HIV/AIDS. *Treatment Issues* July/Aug 1997: 11 (7/8).

Perquin, C.W., A.A.J.M. Hazebroek-Kampschreur, and J.A.M. Hunfeld, et al. Pain in children and adolescents: A common experience. *Pain* 2000; 87: 51–58.

Richlin, D.M. Nonnarcotic analgesics and tricyclic antidepressants for the treatment of chronic nonmalignant pain. *Mt Sinai J Med* 1991; 58: 221–28.

Rosner, H., L. Rubin, and A. Kestenbaum. Gabapentin adjunctive therapy in neuropathic pain states. *Clin J Pain* 1996; 12: 56–58.

Rusy, L.M., and S.J. Weisman. Complementary therapies for acute pediatric pain management. *Pediatr Clin North Am* 2000; 47: 589–99.

Sanfilippo, J.S. Adolscent pelvic pain. *Best Pract Res Clin Obstet Gynaecol* 2003 Feb; 17(1): 93–101.

Sherman, J.J., et al. Effects of stretch-based progressive relaxation training on the secretion of salivary immunoglobulin A in orofacial pain patients. *J Orofac Pain* 1997 Spring 11(2): 115–24.

Silberstein, S.D. Migraine. *Lancet* 2004; 363: 381–91.

Sporrer, K.A., S.M. Jackson, S. Agner, J. Laver, and M.R. Abboud. Pain in children and adolescents with sickle cell anemia: A prospective study utilizing self-reporting. *Am J Pediatr Hematol Oncol* 1994; 16: 219–24.

Stanton-Hicks, M. Reflex sympathetic dystrophy: A sympathetically mediated pain syndrome or not? *Curr Rev Pain* 2000; 4: 268–75.

Stanton-Hicks, M. Complex regional pain syndrome (type I, RSD; type II, causalgia): Controversies. *Clin J Pain* 2000; 16: S33–S40.

Stanton-Hicks, M., R. Baron, R. Boas, T. Gordh, N. Harden, and N. Hendler, et al. Complex regional pain syndromes: Guidelines for therapy. *Clin J Pain* 1998; 14: 155–66.

Taylor, L.M. Complex regional pain syndrome: Comparing adults and adolescents. From Advanced Practice Nursing (eJournal) at www.medscape.com/viewarticle/430537

Tucker, Lori B., M.D. *Your Child with Arthritis: A Family Guide for Caregiving*. Baltimore: Johns Hopkins University Press, 2000.

Varni, J.W., and B.H. Bernstein. Evaluation and management of pain in children with rheumatic diseases. *Rheum Dis Clin North Am* 1991; 17: 985–1000.

Walco, G.A., J.W. Varni, and N.T. Ilowite. Cognitive-behavioral pain management in children with juvenile rheumatoid arthritis. *Pediatrics* 1992; 89: 1075–79.

Wheeler, D.S., K.K. Vaux, and D.A. Tam. Use of gabapentin in the treatment of childhood reflex sympathetic dystrophy. *Pediatr Neurol* 2000; 22: 220–21.

Wilder, R.T., et al. Reflex sympathetic dystrophy in children. Clinical characteristics and follow-up of seventy patients. *J Bone Joint Surg Am* 1992; 74: 910–19.

ASSOCIATIONS/ORGANIZATIONS

American Academy of Orofacial Pain
19 Mantua Road
Mount Royal, NJ 08061
856-423-3629
www.aaop.org

American Chronic Pain Association
PO Box 850
Rocklin, CA 95677-0850
800-533-3231
www.theacpa.org

Amerian Fibromyalgia Syndrome Association
6380 East Tanque Verde, Suite D
Tucson, AZ 85715
520-733-1570
www.afsafund.org

American Massage Therapy Association
820 Davis Street
Evanston, IL 60201
847-864-0123
www.amtamassage.org

American Pain Foundation
201 N. Charles Street, Ste. 710
Baltimore, MD 21201-4111
www.painfoundation.org

Arthritis Foundation
1330 W. Peachtree Street
Atlanta, GA 30309
800-283-7800
www.arthritis.org

Endometriosis Association
8585 N. 76th Place
Milwaukee, WI 53223-2600
800-992-3636
www.endometriosisassn.org

HCG Resources
www.hcgresources.com/resources.html
List of endometriosis resources

National Certification Board for Therapeutic Massage & Bodywork
829 Greensboro Drive, Ste. 300
McLean, VA 22102
1-800-296-0664
www.ncbtmb.com

National Chronic Pain Outreach Association
PO Box 274
Millboro, VA 24460
540-862-9437
www.chronicpain.org

National Foundation for the Treatment of Pain
PO Box 70045
Houston, TX 77270-0045
713-862-9332
www.paincare.org

National Headache Foundation
820 N. Orleans, Ste. 217
Chicago, IL 60610
888-NHF-5552
www.headaches.org

National Pain Foundation
3511 S. Clarkson St.
Englewood, CO 80113
303-783-8899
www.painconnection.org

Reflex Sympathetic Dystrophy Syndrome Association
PO Box 502
Milford, CT 06460
877-662-7737
www.rsds.org

Sinusitis Central
1072 Casitas Pass Road, Ste. 190
Carpinteria, CA 93013
www.sinusitiscentral.com

SUPPORT GROUPS AND ONLINE CHATS

American Council for Headache Education
19 Mantua Road
Mount Royal, NJ 08061
856-423-0258
www.achenet.org
Offers migraine support groups

http://groups.yahoo.com/group/TeenageEndometriosis

American Sickle Cell Anemia Association
Chat room: www.ascao.org/chat.asp

Sickle Cell Disease Association of America

Fibrohugs, monitored chats and forums, information, etc., for people with fibromyalgia, irritable bowel syndrome, migraine, and other similar conditions.
http://fibrohugs.com

Center for Young Women's Health, Children's Hospital Boston
Teens and Endometriosis Chat
www.youngwomenshealth.org/chat.html

PRODUCTS

Relaxation tapes for chronic pain
www.calming.org/pain.htm

LightSeed
PO Box 695
Griswold, CT 06351
888-407-8456
www.lightseed.com/tapes/guided_imagery_emmett_miller.htm

CHILDREN'S HOSPITALS (Alphabetized by State)

Children's Hospital of Alabama
1600 Seventh Avenue South
Birmingham, AL 35233
205-939-9100
www.chsys.org

Phoenix Children's Hospital
1919 E. Thomas Road
Phoenix, AZ 85016
602-546-1000

Arkansas Children's Hospital
800 Marshall Street
Little Rock, AR 72202
501-364-1100
www.archildrens.org

Children's Hospital & Health Center
3020 Children's Way
San Diego, CA 92123
858-576-1700
www.chsd.org

Lucile Salter Packard Children's Hospital at Stanford
725 Welch Road
Palo Alto, CA 94304

650-497-8000
www.lpch.org

Children's Hospital & Research Center
at Oakland
747 52nd Street
Oakland, CA 94609
510-428-3000
www.chodfoundation.org

Children's Hospital of Orange County
455 S. Main Street
Orange, CA 92868
714-997-3000
www.choc.org

Miller Children's Hospital
2801 Atlantic Avenue
Long Beach, CA 90806
562-933-2000

Shriners Hospital for Children, Los Angeles
3160 Geneva Street
Los Angeles, CA 90020
213-388-3151
www.shrinehg.org

Shriners Hospitals for Children,
Northern California
2425 Stockton Boulevard

Sacramento, CA 95817
916-453-2000
www.shrinehg.org

Children's Hospital
1056 East 19th Avenue
Denver, CO 80218
303-861-8888
www.thechildrenshospital.org

Alfred I. duPont Hospital for Children
1600 Rockland Road
Wilmington, DE 19803
302-651-4000
www.nemours.org

Children's National Medical Center
111 Michigan Avenue NW
Washington, DC 20010
202-884-5000
www.cnmc.org

All Children's Hospital
801 Sixth Street South
St. Petersburg, FL
727-898-7451
www.allkids.org

Miami Children's Hospital
3100 SW 62nd Avenue

Miami, FL 33155
305-666-6511
www.mch.com

Children's Healthcare Atlanta
1600 Tollie Circle NE
Atlanta, GA 30329
404-325-6000
www.choa.org

Children's Memorial Hospital
2300 Children's Plaza
Chicago, IL 60614
773-880-4000
www.childrensmemorial.org

Children's Mercy South
5808 West 110th Street
Overland Park, KS 66211
816-234-3653

Children's Hospital
200 Henry Clay Avenue
New Orleans, LA
504-899-9511
www.chnola.org

Children's Hospital Boston
300 Longwood Avenue
Boston, MA 02115

617-355-6000
www.childrenshospital.org

Children's Hospital of Michigan
3901 Beaubien Street
Detroit, MI 48201
313-966-5110
www.chmkids.org

Children's Hospital & Clinics
345 South Smith Avenue
St. Paul, MN 55102
651-220-6000
www.childrenshc.org

Children's Hospitals & Clinics
2525 Chicago Avenue South
Minneapolis, MN 55404
612-813-6100
www.childrenshc.org

Children's Mercy Hospital
2401 Gillham Road
Kansas City, MO 64108
816-234-3000
www.childrens-mercy.org

SSM Cardinal Glennon Children's Hospital
1465 South Grand Boulevard
St. Louis, MO 63104

314-577-5600
www.cardinalglennon.com

St. Louis Children's Hospital
1 Children's Place
St. Louis, MO 63110
314-454-6000
www.stlouischildrens.org

Children's Hospital
8200 Dodge Street
Omaha, NE 68114
402-955-5400
www.chsomaha.org

Akron Children's Hospital
One Perkins Square
Akron, OH 44308
330-543-1000
www.akronchildrens.org

Cincinnati Children's Hospital Medical Center
3333 Burnet Avenue
Cincinnati, OH 45229
www.chmcc.org

Doernbecher Children's Hospital
3181 S.W. Sam Jackson Park Road
Mail Code: DC105

Portland, OR 97201-3098
503-418-5195

Children's Hospital of Philadelphia
34th Street & Civic Center Boulevard
Philadelphia, PA 19104
215-590-7555
www.chop.edu

East Tennessee Children's Hospital
2018 Clinch Avenue
Knoxville, TN 37916
865-541-8000
www.etch.com

Children's Medical Center of Dallas
1935 Motor Street
Dallas, TX 75235
214-456-7000
www.childrens.com

Christus Santa Rosa Children's
Hospital
333 N. Santa Rosa Street
San Antonio, TX 78207
210-704-2011

Cook Children's Medical Center
801 7th Avenue
Ft. Worth, TX 76104

682-885-4000
www.cookchildrens.org

Covenant Children's Hospital
3610 21st Street
Lubbock, TX 79410
806-725-1011
www.covenanthealth.org

Driscoll Children's Hospital
3533 S. Alameda Street
Corpus Christi, TX 78411
361-694-5000
www.driscollchildrens.org

Texas Children's Hospital
6621 Fannin Street
Houston, TX 77030
832-824-1000
www.texaschildrenshospital.org

Primary Children's Medical Center
100 North Medical Drive
Salt Lake City, UT 84113-1100
801-588-2000

Children's Hospital of The Kings
Daughters
601 Children's Lane
Norfolk, VA 23507

757-668-7700
www.chkd.org

Children's Hospital & Regional Medical Center
4800 Sand Point Way NE
Seattle, WA 98105
206-987-2000
www.seattlechildrens.org

Mary Bridge Children's Hospital & Health Center
317 Martin Luther King Jr. Way
Tacoma, WA 98405
253-403-1400
www.multicare.org

Children's Hospital of Wisconsin
9000 W. Wisconsin Avenue
Milwaukee, WI 53226
414-266-2000
www.chw.org

PAIN DIARY

DATE	TIME	PAIN RATING 1-10	MEDS TAKEN (NAME, DOSE)	OTHER THERAPIES	COMMENTS

Index

About the Author

Dr. Elliot Krane was trained in pediatric anesthesia and intensive care at the Harvard Children's Hospital and has devoted the past twenty years to refining and innovating techniques, strategies, and therapies to relieve the suffering of children with chronic pain. For nearly ten years he has been a Professor of Pediatrics and a Professor of Anesthesia at Stanford University School of Medicine and since 2001 has been the director of Pain Therapeutics, Inc., a multidisciplinary pediatric pain clinic at Lucile Packard Children's Hospital in San Francisco. He has lectured internationally on the topic of pediatric pain management and has been widely published in professional journals.